Essays in the History

of Nephrology

Essays in the History of Nephrology

Robert I. Levy, MD

Studies in Medicine, History and Culture

Volume 2

Series Editor: David B. Levy, PhD

2018

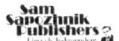
Sam
Sanczhnik
Publishers
Fiercely Independent

To my parents

Robert I. Levy, MD
and
Ruth S. Levy, ה"ע

Studies in Medicine, History and Culture

Volume One

Music and Medicine

Volume Two

Essays in The History of Nephrology

Volume Three

Essays in History of Medicine

Volume Four

Essays in the History of Allied Sciences

Volume Five

Pierre Rayer's *Treatise sur Les Reins:* A New Translation

Series Editor: David B. Levy, PhD

Preface

Robert I. Levy's first interest in the history of medicine was in high school in 1941 with a paper on the History of Anesthesia. He remembers visiting the Welch Library at the Johns Hopkins Medical School for the first time and entering the stacks in search of some material. Dr Levy had the opportunity to visit the Massachusetts General Hospital and the opportunity of visiting the Ether Dome in the Bullfinch Building where anesthesia was first presented in 1950.

In the Johns Hopkins Medical School Dr. Levy had the opportunity to work part time in the lab of Department of Medicine under Drs. Joseph Lillenthal and Kenneth Zieler. This was a wonderful learning experience developing laboratory technique and produced three papers with his name using Warburg apparatus to study metabolism of rat diaphragm, published in the *Bulletin of the Johns Hopkins Hospital* in 1953. (see bibliography)

While a fellow in the Pharmacology Department of the Johns Hopkins Medical School in 1956-58 with Dr. Gilbert Mudge he worked on the metabolism of diuretics in dogs. This produced two papers published in *the Journal of Clinical Investigation* in 1958 and 1962. (see bibliography)

As a Resident in Medicine at the Sinai Hospital in Baltimore he dialysed a patient on a Kolff Twin Coil Kidney with ethylene glycol poisoning in 1958 and wrote up the experience published in *the Journal of the American Medical Association* in 1960. (see bibliography) This was one of the first patients dialysed in Baltimore before the procedure was performed at Hopkins Hospital later.

Additional review articles were published when Dr. Levy first went into practice of medicine in the *Sinai Hospital Journal* in 1961 on "Steroid blocking agents as diuretic agents," and in 1962 on "Serum sodium concentration, Facts and Fancy" in *the Indian Medical Journal* in 1962, and "Antibiotics and "Digitalis Administration in Uremia" as an editorial in *the Maryland Medical Journal* 13, 35, 1964.

As a result of working in the lab of the Department of Medicine on a NIH grant on Lipids in the Nephrotic syndrome, Dr Levy published a paper in *the fifteenth Annual Conference on the Kidney in* 1964. (see Bibliography)

In 1964 working with a medical student, Dr. Stewart Fine, who eventually became Head of the Ophthalmology Department at University of Pennsylvania, there was published in *the New England Journal of Medicine* one of the first articles on treatment of pulmonary edema with a then newly released diuretic, Ethacrynic Acid, labeled as a "bloodless phlebotomy."

Again early in his practice Dr. Levy published an article in 1966, "Studies in a Patient with Chyluria" published in *the Journal of Clinical Nutrition*. Also a study of "Overwhelming Salicylate intoxication in an Adult published in 1967 in *the Archives of Internal Medicine*. (see bibliography) Both of these papers grew out of clinical presentations, chyluria and salicylate intoxication.

Additional papers were published on the treatment of hypercalcemia, with forced saline diuresis and Ethacrynic Acid, a study in dogs and a review of "the Clinical Spectrum of Lactic Acidosis." (see bibliography)

Further papers on Bromide Detection and Diagnosis of Bromism from the laboratory standpoint and a paper on Ectopic ACTH and Hpernatremia were published. (see bibliography)

The presentation of a patient with chyloperitoneum on peritoneal dialysis, presented an opportunity to publish in *the American Journal of Kidney Diseases* in 2001, a paper on studies on this patient and the use of medium chain triglyercide (MCT oil) in this patient. (see bibliography)

After Dr Levy's retirement from the practice of medicine. Dr. Levy then [as well as continuing bikur holim visits], began devoting his leisure to exploring topics in the history of medicine by doing research in the library of the History of Medicine at Hopkins. Since then Dr. Levy regularly presents papers to *the American Osler Society* as well as in other forums such as the American Urological Association (paper on Homer Smith). With a long experience in the practice of nephrology Dr Levy started out on evaluating certain aspects of the History of Nephrology.

The first of these papers on the History of Nephrology was entitled "The Reception in Britain and on the Continent of Richard Bright's *Reports of Medical Cases Linking Dropsy, Coagualable Urine and Small Granular Kidneys as a Clinical Entity- Edinburg, Dublin and Paris.*" This paper discusses not only the work of Richard Bright but those who followed, Robert Christian in Scotland,

Jonathan Osborn in Dublin, Ireland, and Pierre Rayer in Paris.

The next paper *A Garland of Ibids: The use of Footnotes in the Medical Writings of Early Nineteenth Century Authors who Established Bright's Disease as a Clinical Entity"* reviews the use of the extensive footnotes used in the above author's writings.

Next in the series of papers on the History of Nephrology is a paper entitled, *The Urinalysis as a Factor in the Establishment of the Clinical Entity of Bright's Disease in the Early 19th Century.* This paper discusses the discovery of urea by Von Rouelle and its further purification and characterization by Fourcroy and Vauquelin who called it *uree.* Berzellus, William Prout, John Bostock, George Owen Ress, and the Animal Chemists in the Circle of Richard Bright are discussed.

The Animal chemists in the Circle of Richard Bright is a further paper describing the contributions to better understanding renal disease by the work of Berzelius, von Liebig in Germany and Bostock, Prout, Reese, Babington, Barlow and Mr. Tweedies, and in France, Fourcroy and Dumas.

The Therapeutic Spectrum Available to Those Defining a Newly Recognized Clinical Entity—Bright's Disease discusses the multiple plant sources for medication.

The paper *Pulvis Ipecacunanhae et Opii—The Powder and the Buccaneer—Thomas Dover* further discusses the use of medication available to the early physicians carrying for patients with Bright's Disease.

A Conversation Between Two Leeches is a comic attempt at humor to discuss leeches in the therapy of renal disease as well as their wide spread use in the past.

A miscellaneous group of papers followed, the next two having to do with William Osler presented to the Osler society, to give a more balanced view of his "therapeutic nihilism:

Sir William Osler's View on Pierre C.A. Louis' Recommendations for Bleeding in Pneumonia—Paradox of Calling his Method Iconoclastic.

Sir William Olser—Departure from his Reputation as a Therapeutic Conservative—The Treatment of Bright's Disease.

PAPERS IN HISTORY OF MEDICINE AND MEDICAL HUMANITIES

Dr Levy presented the following paper on *The Doctor and the Newspaper Editor/Correspondence between Logan Clendening, M.D. and H.L. Mencken* at the request of the Medical Department of the University of Kansas Medical School. Logan Clendening, M.D. was known to have been influenced by H. L Menckin in initiating his writing career but little else was known about the relationship. Dr. Levy was a fan of H.L. Mencken, having heard him speak while he was in high school and is a member of the Mencken Society. The paper is the result of Dr Levy's archival search at the Enoch Pratt Library and Goucher Collage Libraries in Baltimore. It covers not only the occasion of their initial meeting and suggestions of Mencken on writing, but a twenty-two year additional follow up friendship that covered a variety of subjects.

The History of Sinai Hospital was suggested to Dr. Levy by the Chief of Medicine at the Sinai Hospital in Baltimore. While Dr. Levy was born at the Sinai Hospital and was a chief resident in medicine as well as practicing at this hospital for over forty years, the history of the Hospital from its founding in 1863, the third oldest Jewish Hospital in America, was very little appreciated. It is hoped this paper will bring to light the significance and and history of Sinai Hospital in Baltimore.

Colour Indicator, Robert Boyle's *Experimental History of Colours and Lignum nephritcum* was a tale of the Spanish explorers bringing back to the Old World a wood from a tree that produced a blue color, when clear water was placed on it, and was considered by the Mexican Indians and the Old World when it was brought back to Europe in the middle of the 16th Century to treat kidney diseases for over 400 years. Robert Boyle however used it to formulate a definition of acids and bases that was an early advance in modern chemistry. This blue color was also the first known example of fluorescence, a concept not identified until the 19th Century.

PAPERS IN MUSIC AND MEDICINE

Mozart and Medicine at the end of the 18th Century

Johannes Brahms and Dr. Theodor Billroth: A Musical Friendship of the composer and the surgeon

Musicians of the High Baroque, Johann Sebastian Bach and George Frideric Handel and the State of Opthamology in the 17th and 18th Centuries

Many other papers were written such as:

Homer Smith and the evolution of the Kidney (presented at the American Urological Association)

William August Marburg's relationship with Sir William Osler

William Harvey's De Motu Cordis

John Conrad Hemmeter, Gastroenterologist: A Tribute to a Historian of Medicine and Science

Book review in *the Journal of the History of Medicine and Allied Science*s on the History of Nephrology 4: Reports from the Third Congress of the International Association for the History of Nephrology, Basel Switzerland, S. Karger AG 2002 vi, 218 illus. cloth, etc.

"Bubbles appearing on the surface of the urine indicate disease of the kidneys and a prolonged illness... colorless urine is bad... the sudden appearance of blood in the urine indicates that a small renal vessel has burst"

(Hippocrates, Corpus Hippocraticum)

"The living organism does not really exist in the milieu exterieur (the atmosphere if it breathes, salt or fresh water if that is its element) but in the liquid milieu interieur formed by circulating organic liquid, which surrounds and bathes all tissue elements... the stability of the milieu interieur is the primary condition for freedom and independence of existence, the mechanism which allows this is that which ensures in the milieu interieur the maintenance of all conditions necessary to the life of the elements."

(Claude Bernard)

Neither the urea clearance nor any other physiological measurement should be asked to serve as the sole criterion to be discriminated between health and disease. The clinician using such a test must evaluate the results in terms of all known causes of variation, physiological and pathological.

(Donald Van Slyke, 1949)

"A patient needs a doctor not a committee.. Doctors treat individuals, not statistical averages... If you don't examine the trees, you may get lost in the woods. The proper study of mankind is man."

(John P Peters MD)

The responsibility for maintaining the composition of the blood in respect to other constituents devolves largely upon the kidneys. It is no exaggeration to say that the composition of the blood is determined not by what the mouth ingests but by what the kidneys keep; they are the master chemists of our internal environment, which, so to speak, they synthesize in reverse. When, among other duties, they excrete the ashes of our body fires, or remove from the blood the infinite variety of foreign substances which are constantly being absorbed from our indiscriminate gastrointestinal tracts, these excretory operations are incidental to the major task of keeping our internal environment in an ideal, balanced state. Our glands, our muscles, our bones, our tendons, even our brains, are called upon to do only one kind of physiological work, while our kidneys are called upon to perform an innumerable variety of operations. Bones can break, muscles can atrophy, glands can loaf, even the brain can go to sleep, without immediately endangering our survival, but when the kidneys fail to manufacture the proper kind of blood neither bone, muscle, gland nor brain can carry on.

(Homer Smith, 'The Evolution of the Kidney', *Lectures on the Kidney* (1943), 3

There are those who say that the human kidney was created to keep the blood pure, or more precisely, to keep our internal environment in an ideal balanced state.... I contend that the human kidney manufactures the kind of urine that it does, and it maintains the blood in the composition which that fluid has, because this kidney has a certain functional architecture; and it owes that architecture not to design or foresight or to any plan, but to the fact that the earth is an unstable sphere with a fragile crust, to the geologic revolutions that for six hundred million years have raised and lowered continents and seas, to the predacious enemies, and heat and cold, and storms and droughts; to the unending succession of vicissitudes that have driven the mutant vertebrates from sea into fresh water, into desiccated swamps, out upon the dry land, from one habitation to another, perpetually in search of the free and independent life, perpetually failing, for one reason or another, to find it.

(Homer Smith, From Fish To Philosopher, (1953), 210-1.)

To accuse another of having weak kidneys, lungs, or heart is not a crime; on the contrary saying he has a week brain is a crime.

(Primo Levi)

Biblical & Rabbinic Citations to the Kidneys
(Reins)

אֲבָרֵךְ—אֶת- ד',
אֲשֶׁר יְעָצָנִי;
אַף-לֵילוֹת, יִסְּרוּנִי
כִלְיוֹתָי.

7 I will bless the LORD, who hath given me counsel; yea, in the night seasons my reins instruct me (yisserun)

(Psalm 16:7)

Examine me O Lord and prove me, try my reins and my heart / (צָרְפָה) צרופה   בְּחָנֵנִי ד' וְנַסֵּנִי;
כִלְיוֹתַי וְלִבִּי
(Psalms 26:2)

כִּי-אַתָּה, קָנִיתָ כִלְיֹתָי; תְּסֻכֵּנִי, בְּבֶטֶן אִמִּי.

13 For Thou hast made my reins; Thou hast knit me together in my mother's womb.

(Psalm 139:13)

I the Lord search the heart; I try the reins, even to give every man according to his ways and according to the fruit of his doings / אֲנִי ד' חֹקֵר לֵב, בֹּחֵן כְּלָיוֹת: וְלָתֵת לְאִישׁ כִּדְרָכָו, כִּפְרִי מַעֲלָלָיו

(Jeremiah 17:10)

וְהָיָה צֶדֶק, אֵזוֹר מָתְנָיו; וְהָאֱמוּנָה, אֵזוֹר חֲלָצָיו.

5 And righteousness shall be the girdle of his loins, and faithfulness the girdle of his reins

(Isaiah 11:5)

לֹו מִי-שָׁת, בַּטֻּחוֹת חָכְמָה; אוֹ מִי-נָתַן לַשֶּׂכְוִי בִינָה.

36 Who hath put wisdom in the inward parts? Or who hath given understanding to the mind?

(Job 38:36)

טו בְּנִי, אִם-חָכַם לִבֶּךָ-- יִשְׂמַח לִבִּי גַם-אָנִי.

15 My son, if thy heart be wise, my heart will be glad, even mine;

טז וְתַעְלֹזְנָה   **16** Yea, my reins will
כִלְיוֹתָי--   בְּדַבֵּר   rejoice, when thy lips
שְׂפָתֶיךָ, מֵישָׁרִים.   speak right things.

(Mishlei 28:6)

קהלת רבה (וילנא) פרשה ז:
מעשרה שליטים שמשמשין את הנפש, ואלו הן, הוושט למזון,
קנה לקול, כבד לחמה, מרה לקנאה, הריאה מששתן, המסס
לטחון, טחול לשחוק כליות יועצות, לב מבין, לשון גומר.

The kidneys give advice (kelayot yo'azot), the heart
comprehends (mevin), the tongue articulated (literally
cuts), and the mouth concludes (gomer) Hullin 11a;
Shabbat 33b, Koheleth Rabbati 7:36; Avot de Rabbi
Nathan 31:3

בראשית רבה (וילנא) פרשת חיי שרה פרשה סא
כי אם בתורת ה' חפצו, כי ידעתיו למען אשר יצוה, ובתורתו
יהגה אר"ש אב לא למדו ורב לא היה לו, ומהיכן למד את
התורה, אלא זימן לו הקב"ה שתי כליותיו כמין שני רבנים
והיו נובעות ומלמדות אותו תורה וחכמה, הה"ד (תהלים טז)
אברך את ה' אשר יעצני אף לילות יסרוני כליותי,
(שם /תהלים/ א) והיה כעץ שתול ששתלו הקב"ה בארץ
ישראל, אשר פריו יתן בעתו זה ישמעאל ועלהו לא יבול זה
יצחק, וכל אשר יעשה יצליח אלו בני קטורה שנאמר ויוסף
אברהם ויקח אשה

Table of Contents

Introduction
Historical Overview of the History of Nephrology

David B Levy (PhD; MLS)

From the table of contents the reader can see that most of the essays included in this volume treat developments in the history of nephology from the 18th, 19th, and 20th centuries. However it should be noted that medical knowledge of the kidneys extends from antiquity, much earlier than modernity, although the field of nephrology may be a construct of modern making. This is apparent from the classification of the table of contents of a work like Julius Preuss' classic, *Biblical and Talmudic Medicine,* that organizes ancient and medieval medical and folk medicine ideas and opinions, within the rubric and architectonic of modern medical sub disciplines.

While Osler gave us the assignment to trace an evolution of Modern Medicine[1] we must do detective work to uncover the medicine of antiquity and the medieval periods. Let us consider very briefly in this introduction some views of the significance of the kidneys and aspects associated with them in antiquity forward to the

---

[1] Osler, William, The Evolution of Modern Medicine, New Haven: Yale Univ. Press, 1921

Renaissance.[2] From the Bible,[3] Talmudim,[4] and Midrashim we hope to illustrate that the kidneys: (1) are considered the most remote, innermost, hidden, and mysterious of all the human organs enveloped in mystery and secrets, (2) they (associated with counsel and advice) are related to the heart which understands, being a kind of counterpart working in tandem in the lower part of the person, and (3) they are not only the seat of counsel and advice but of feeling, perhaps even moral consciousness according to Rabbi Avraham ibn Ezra and thus the source of instruction of Torah to Avraham.

Medicine and Kidneys from Bible[5] to Talmud[6]- How the kelayot came to be associated with Aitzah (advice)

Statistical note on Number of times Kidneys mentioned and Health in the Bible

---

[2] Black D., *J R Soc Med* 1980 Jul;73(7):514-8. The story of nephrology;

[3] Gordon, BL, Medicine among the ancient Hebrews. Ann Med Hist 4, 219-235, 1942; Allan, N, The Physican in ancient Israel, His status and function, Med Hist 45, 377-394, 2001; Gordon, MB, Medicine among the ancient Hebrew, ISIS 33: 454-485, 1941

[4] See Snowman, J: A Short History of Talmudic Medicine, New York: Hermon Press, 1973 and Preuss, J, Biblische und Talmudische Medicin;Dvorjetski, E, The History of nephrology in the Talmudic Corpus, Am J Nephrology 22: 119-129, 2002

[5] Koppel, JD, the Biblcal view of the kidney, Am J Neprhology 14:279-281, 1994

[6] See Rosner, Fred, The Encyclopedia of Medicine in the Bible and Talmud, Northvale, NJ, Jason Aronson Inc. 2000

The Kidneys are mentioned in twenty six verses in the Hebrew Bible always in the plural (kelayot).[7] Eleven times mention of the kidneys is with regards to sacrifices in the Jerusalem Temple.[8] The use in the plural suggests that in the time of the Bible it was known there are two kidneys. Knowledge of the existence of two kidneys in Rabbinic thought suggested to the rabbis that there are in humans two forces, one to give good and the other bad advice.[9]

In the Humash they are cited eleven times regarding the korbanot (sacrifices). Often Sacrifices were seen as divine theurgic action to ward off medical illness. According to Josephus sacrificial offerings were made for the expulsion of disease.[10]

In Jeremiah and Psalms the Kidneys are cited metaphorically as the location of temperament, emotions, prudence, vigor and wisdom.

---

[7] *Tuhot* is also used for kidneys in the Bible in Iyov 38:36 "Who has put wisdom (hokmah) in the inward parts (tuhot)?" . The midrash asks "how do we know that these tuhot are the kidneys? Because they are wedged (or squeezed- tuah) in the body. The etymology of tuhot is kidneys because they are wedged between other organs. It is implied that knowledge is stored in the kidneys. The Talmud does use the single form kolya, kolyitha several times. The Hebrew *kelayot* is rendered in Aramaic in the Talmud and Targumim by *kolyan*, the plural of *kolya*.

[8] Cf Ex 29:13; 29:22; Lev 3:4; 3:10;3:15; 4:9; 7:4; 8:15; 9:10; 9:19

[9] Kottek, SS: "The kidneys give advice"- Some thoughts on nephrology in the Talmud and Midrash, in Korot 10, 44-53, 1994

[10] Josephus, Jewish Antiquities Book III, Cambridge, Loeb Classical Library, Harvard Univ Press, p.429-431, 2001

In five instances the kidneys are mentioned as the loci that God examines to judge a person. In Jeremiah 17:10 God is said to search the heart and kidneys:

אֲנִי ד' חֹקֵר לֵב, בֹּחֵן כְּלָיוֹת: וְלָתֵת לְאִישׁ כִּדְרָכָו, כִּפְרִי מַעֲלָלָיו. {ס}	**10** I the LORD search the heart, I try the reins, even to give every man according to his ways, according to the fruit of his doings.

This idea is further found in Psalms 26:2

בְּחָנֵנִי ד' וְנַסֵּנִי; צרופה (צָרְפָה) כִלְיוֹתַי וְלִבִּי.	**2** Examine me, O LORD, and try me; test my reins and my heart.

All five mentions of this searching and testing the hidden organs of the heart and kidney are in Jeremiah and Psalms. This idea perhaps suggests that the heart and kidneys are the key essence of a person

There is also reference to the kidneys as the site of divine punishment for sins particularly in the book of Iyov (Job). We are told that "if only we would hearken to the voice of the L-rd and follow His statutes and commandments then G-d will not put any of the diseases upon them, which He has put upon the Egyptians "for I am the L-rd that health thee" (Ex 15:26).

Divine injury to the kidneys is mentioned three times. Job laments:

יָסֹבּוּ עָלַי,
רַבָּיו -- יְפַלַּח
כִּלְיוֹתַי, וְלֹא
יַחְמֹל;
יִשְׁפֹּךְ לָאָרֶץ,
מְרֵרָתִי.

13 His archers compass me round about, He cleaveth my reins asunder, and doth not spare; He poureth out my gall upon the ground

Again Job protests:

אֲשֶׁר אֲנִי,
אֶחֱזֶה-לִּי--וְעֵינַי
רָאוּ וְלֹא-זָר:
כָּלוּ כִלְיֹתַי
בְּחֵקִי.

27 Whom I, even I, shall see for myself, and mine eyes shall behold, and not another's. My reins are consumed within me.

Jeremiah similarly says:

הֵבִיא,
בְּכִלְיוֹתָי, בְּנֵי,
אַשְׁפָּתוֹ.

13 He hath caused the arrows of His quiver to enter into my reins

We can only surmise that injury to the kidneys as divine retribution was thought by the biblical audience to causes kidney disease.

In the surrounding culture of Ancient Mesopotamia[11] it was often felt, as in the medieval ages that illness was attributed to possession by demons and bad spirits.[12] Illness was sometimes perceived as punishment for transgressions against divinities or breached promises.[13] Rambam condemned such superstitions and forbid incantations, spells, and prayers to be recited over wounds or to remove the cause of disease to cure it directly.[14]

The Biblical View of medicine and the kidneys

The Biblical view considered the kidneys, like the heart associated with mystery, in that they are hidden organs deep in the body but accessible by the penetrating sight of God. Josephus attributes to King Solomon a great wisdom of medical knowledge.[15] Legend has it that Solomon compiled a book of remedies that was

---

[11] Dawson, WR: Clio Meica: The Beginnings: Egypt and Assyria, NY, Paul B Hoeber, Inc. 1930

[12] As this relates to mental illness see Foucault, Michel, Madness and Civilization, NY: Vintage Books, 1965

[13] Jastrow, M., The medicine of Babylonians and Assyrians, Proc Royal Sco Medicine 7, 109-176,1914; also see Geller MJ, Die babylonysch-assyriche Medizin in Texten und Untersuchungen 7 in Renal and Rectal Disease texts, Berlin Walter de Gruyten GMBH & Co. 2005; Jayne WA, The Healing gods of Ancient Civilizations, New Haven: Yale Univ Press 1925

[14] See Strickman, Norman, Without red strings or holy water: Maimonides' Mishneh Torah, Brighton MA: Academic Studies Press, 2011

[15] Josephus, Jewish Wars, Book VII, Cambridge, Loeb Classical Library: Harvard Univ. Press, 2001

subsequently found and concealed by Hezekiah.[16] Solomon's wisdom is said to have excelled the wisdom of all the children of the east country and all of the wisdom of Egypt (I Kings 4:29). Before Solomon, Moses had instructed a bronze serpent named *Nehushtan* to be erected to relieve the effects of a plague of poisonous snakes (Num. 21:8-9). A copy was later placed in the Jerusalem *Beit HaMikdash* until Hezekiah took it down and destroyed it because he felt it was idolatrous (2 Kgs 18:4). However the Greek *cadeusus*, the symbol of many medical associations, seems to derive from this more ancient tradition.[17]

The first mention of the word physician or healer in the Bibe is in Genesis 50:2 were Joseph employs a physician to embalm his father Yakov Avinu. It is well known amongst scholars of Egyptology[18] that in the mummification process the kidneys[19] were extracted and embalmed in a solution that would preserve them and then reset in the body cavity. [20]

---

[16] See Gordon, BL, Medicine among the ancient Hebrews. Ann Med Hist 4: 219-235, 1942; Allan N.: The physician in ancient Israel. His status and function. Med History 45, 377-394, 2001

[17] Schouten J, The Road and the Serpent of Asklepios, Symbol of Medicine, Amsterdam: Elsevier Pub Co, 1967

[18] Smith, GE Heart and reins in mummification, J Manchester Univ Egyptian Oriental Soc 1, 41-44, 1911; Leca A., The Egyptian way of Death, Mummies and the Cult of the Immortal, Garden City: NY Doubleday and Co., 1981, p. 144-146

[19] Salem, ME Eknoyan G, The kidney in ancient Egyptian medicine, Where does it stand? Am J Nephrology 19, 140-147, 1999

[20] Budge EAW, The Egyptian Book of the Dead The Papyrus of Ani, NY: Dover Pub, 1967

Kidneys and Korbanot

Eleven times the kidneys are offered up in sacrifices to be burned in the Temple offerings. In Exodus we read;

וְלָקַחְתָּ, אֶת-כָּל-הַחֵלֶב הַמְכַסֶּה אֶת-הַקֶּרֶב, וְאֵת הַיֹּתֶרֶת עַל-הַכָּבֵד, וְאֵת שְׁתֵּי הַכְּלָיֹת וְאֶת-הַחֵלֶב אֲשֶׁר עֲלֵיהֶן; וְהִקְטַרְתָּ, הַמִּזְבֵּחָה.

13 And thou shalt take all the fat that covereth the inwards, and the lobe above the liver, and the two kidneys, and the fat that is upon them, and make them smoke upon the altar.

Aaron makes sacrifice of the kidneys in Deut 32:14 where we learn:

יד חֶמְאַת בָּקָר וַחֲלֵב צֹאן, עִם-חֵלֶב כָּרִים וְאֵילִים   בְּנֵי-בָשָׁן וְעַתּוּדִים, עִם-חֵלֶב, כִּלְיוֹת חִטָּה;   וְדַם-עֵנָב, תִּשְׁתֶּה-חָמֶר

The kidney fat was considered some of the best that could be offered to God as only the best and most fit was appropriate in sacrifices. In fact if the kidneys were deformed or deficient they were not fit (roy) to be brought on the altar. The blades used for sacrifice were considered holy and blessed and related in some way to the success of Israeli troops over enemies. Thus we learn in Isaiah 34:6

חֶרֶב לד' מָלְאָה
דָם, הֻדַּשְׁנָה מֵחֵלֶב,
מִדַּם כָּרִים
וְעַתּוּדִים, מֵחֵלֶב
כִּלְיוֹת אֵילִים: כִּי
זֶבַח לד' בְּבָצְרָה,
וְטֶבַח גָּדוֹל בְּאֶרֶץ
אֱדוֹם.

6 The sword of the LORD is filled with blood, it is made fat with fatness, with the blood of lambs and goats, with the fat of the kidneys of rams; for the LORD hath a sacrifice in Bozrah, and a great slaughter in the land of Edom.

Bible and the Kidneys: Hygiene[21]

The Bible as the work of Julius Preuss (Biblical and Talmudic Medicine) shows, contains many references to medical subjects, that consist of laws governing personal and social cleanliness. In the Bible hygiene is viewed as leading to the prevention of diseases and prophylaxis and ensures individual and community safety as a public health consideration. The children of Israel wandered for forty years in the desert living in close proximity to each other. The potential for outbreaks of contagion and epidemics were real dangers. Thus strict rules of hygiene were required in the desert to prevent epidemics. The bible provides rules for cleanliness of dermetology, garments, dwelling and lodging, and foodstuffs and provides guidelines to prevent the spread of contagion via quarantine.

Statement of Pinchas ben Yair from Avodah Zarah, that adorns opening of Ramhal's Mesilat Yesharim,

21 Omran, AR: The epidemiology transition: A Theory of the epidemiology of population change. Milbank Mem Fund Q 49: 509-538, 1971

that affirms importance of cleanliness (hygiene both physical and spiritual):

R. Pinchas ben Yair once said:
"Torah leads to Watchfulness;
Watchfulness leads to Zeal;
Zeal leads to Cleanliness;
Cleanliness leads to Separation;
Separation leads to Purity;
Purity leads to Saintliness;
Saintliness leads to Humility;
Humility leads to Fear of Sin;
Fear of Sin leads to Holiness;
Holiness leads to the Holy Spirit,
and the Holy Spirit leads to the Revival of the Dead."

--Avodah Zara 20b

From Julius Preuss' *Biblisch-talmudische Medizin* (1923) and M. Perlmann's *Midrash ha-Refu'ah*, [3 vols. (1926–34)] we learn In the Bible Lepers (persons with dermatological uncleanness), anyone who had an "issue," and all who were polluted by contact with a corpse, were excluded from the limits of the camp for specific periods of quarantineLev. 15:1–15; Num. 5:1–4: Persons who touched a carcass, a creeping animal, or a reptile were similarly "defiled," as were the vessels into which these objects might have fallen (Lev. 11:27–40). The Bible also stresses the cleanliness of garments (Eccles. 9:8). The rabbis ordained that one must wash one's face, hands, and feet daily in honor of one's Maker (Shab. 50b).[22] The hands must also be washed on certain occasions: after rising from bed in the morning, after urination and/or defecation, bathing, clipping of the fingernails, removal of shoes, touching the naked foot, washing the hair, visiting a cemetery, touching a corpse, undressing, sexual intercourse, touching a louse, or touching any part of the body generally clothed (Sh. Ar., OH 4:18). It is a particularly important religious duty to wash hands before eating a meal (Hul. 105a–b; Sh. Ar., OH 158–165). Similarly, hands should be washed after the meal and before grace (*mayim aharonim*), because, inadvertently, a person may touch his eyes with salty hands (Hul. *ibid.*) A kohen may not pronounce the priestly benediction if his hands are soiled (Meg. 24b). No prayer may be recited by one who is in a state of physical uncleanliness, or about to relieve himself, or has touched parts of his body generally covered by clothing, without either washing his hands, or rubbing them in sand (Sh. Ar., OH 92:1, 4, 6). In mishnaic times, it was forbidden to drink any liquid (water, wine, milk) which was left uncovered overnight, lest it had been defiled by a venomous snake (Ter. 8:4; Sh. Ar., YD 116:1), and the *Gemara* advised that all foodstuffs be protected from flies because they may have been in contact with persons suffering from skin diseases (Ket. 77b). The rabbis also stressed the importance of public health. The Talmud rules that no carcass, grave, or tannery be placed within 50 ells of a human dwelling (BB 2:9), and insisted that streets and market places be kept clean (Yal. 184). In Jerusalem, they were swept daily (BM 26a). Scholars were forbidden to live in a

---

[22] *Encyclopaedia Judaica*, "Hygiene."

city in which there was no doctor or where there was no bathhouse (Sanh. 17b). Hillel the Elder considered that the act of bathing is an act of caring for the vessel containing the divine spirit (Lev. R. 34:3). Yet as always practical the rabbis conceptualized ways of purification from uncleanliness such as immersion in a mikveh, an subject which Yonatan Adler has written about in an article on "the Origins of Tevilah." On 4/26/18 168 hits appear to scholarly peer reviewed articles regarding immersion in a mikveh with regards to laws of purity. The parah adamah (red cow) is another area whereby the ashes of this animal have the power to purify one from contact with a corpse. Twelve tractates of the Talmud organized around the sixth section of the Mishnah called Tohorot ("Purities"), pertain to the laws of purity and impurity, including the impurity of the dead, the laws of food purity and bodily purity.

In Exodus 19:10 we read of the need for washing garments:

וַיֹּאמֶר ד' אֶל-מֹשֶׁה **10** And the LORD said unto
לֵךְ אֶל-הָעָם, Moses: 'Go unto the people, and
וְקִדַּשְׁתָּם הַיּוֹם sanctify them to-day and to-
וּמָחָר; וְכִבְּסוּ, morrow, and let them wash their
שִׂמְלֹתָם. garments,

In Deuteronomy 23:10-14 rules for military hygiene are given:

כִּי-תֵצֵא מַחֲנֶה, עַל-אֹיְבֶיךָ: וְנִשְׁמַרְתָּ--מִכֹּל, דָּבָר רָע.

10 When thou goest forth in camp against thine enemies, then thou shalt keep thee from every evil thing.

יא כִּי-יִהְיֶה בְךָ אִישׁ, אֲשֶׁר לֹא-יִהְיֶה טָהוֹר מִקְּרֵה-לָיְלָה--וְיָצָא אֶל-מִחוּץ לַמַּחֲנֶה, לֹא יָבֹא אֶל-תּוֹךְ הַמַּחֲנֶה.

11 If there be among you any man, that is not clean by reason of that which chanceth him by night, then shall he go abroad out of the camp, he shall not come within the camp.

יב וְהָיָה לִפְנוֹת-עֶרֶב, יִרְחַץ בַּמָּיִם; וּכְבֹא הַשֶּׁמֶשׁ, יָבֹא אֶל-תּוֹךְ הַמַּחֲנֶה.

12 But it shall be, when evening cometh on, he shall bathe himself in water; and when the sun is down, he may come within the camp.

יג וְיָד תִּהְיֶה לְךָ, מִחוּץ לַמַּחֲנֶה; וְיָצָאתָ שָּׁמָּה, חוּץ.

13 Thou shalt have a place also without the camp, whither thou shalt go forth abroad.

In Leviticus hygiene of food is urged as a preventive against disease:

זֹאת תּוֹרַת הַבְּהֵמָה, וְהָעוֹף, וְכֹל נֶפֶשׁ הַחַיָּה, הָרֹמֶשֶׂת בַּמָּיִם; וּלְכָל-נֶפֶשׁ, הַשֹּׁרֶצֶת עַל-הָאָרֶץ.

46 This is the law of the beast, and of the fowl, and of every living creature that moveth in the waters, and of every creature that swarmeth upon the earth;

מז לְהַבְדִּיל, בֵּין
הַטָּמֵא וּבֵין הַטָּהֹר;
וּבֵין הַחַיָּה,
הַנֶּאֱכֶלֶת, וּבֵין
הַחַיָּה, אֲשֶׁר לֹא
{תֵאָכֵל. פ}

47 to make a difference
between the unclean and the
clean, and between the living
thing that may be eaten and
the living thing that may not
be eaten.

The prohibition of not eating pork, is not just to prevent trichinosis, but that the pig was considered unclean, in that it eats excrement and wallows in filth. Further the pig was thought to represent "hypocrisy" because it would hold out its cloven hooves (a mark of kashrut) but it does not chew its cud. This asymmetry to the animal kingdom taxonomy and classification that most cloven footed animals chew their cud (i.e. deer) seemed to be an anomaly that perhaps the Biblical authority viewed as a disjunction in the order of the naturally established order of the animal kingdom, like plowing with a mule and ox, or hybrids known as kelayim such as grafting plants and trees together, mixing genetic order, or breeding animals of different classifications, or mixing fruits through genetic engineering? Thus perhaps the pig represented a kind of tampering with G-d's design because it has cloven hooves and should be expected to chew its cud, but does not? Blending different species is seen as unnatural tampering with G-d's perfect naturally created ordered and highly designed world.[23]

In Jewish law consumption of blood is also prohibited because in the blood resides the soul of the animal (Lev 7:11).

---

[23] The question may arise, as it did for a Roman opponent to brit milah, "If G-d's natural world is perfect, why must Jewish babies be circumcised?" There are many coherent answers to this polemic. One interprets the foreskin as a defect. Many physicians understand this in part in arguing that the foreskin, if not removed, leaves room for uncleanliness and many urological and dermatological problems. Some Rabbinic commentaries thus deduce that *oral*, the possession of a foreskin, as a physical defect, and circumcision as an act of healing or perfection. The question arises why did G-d command Avraham to circumcise Yitzchak on the 8th day, eight being a symbolic number for what is beyond nature (memalah li-tevah). One response is that the organ of procreation be beyond the realm of animal instinct and in the service of G-d to bring into being children raised with Torah ethics. Genesis 17 does not give reasons for hygiene which are logically deductible, but rather commands that circumcision is a sign of the covenant. We learn in Genesis 17:11 ונמלתם את בשר ערלתכם, והיה לאות ברית ביני וביניכם. In Gen Rabbah 11:6 a reason is given for Brit Milah. A philosopher asked Rabbi Hoshaya "If circumcision is so valued, why wasn't it given to the first man?" [i.e. why wasn't Adam born circumcised] He said to him: "...Anything created on the first six days of creation needs some work. Mustard seeds need sweetening; lupine needs sweetening; grain needs to be ground. Even humans require correction." Further in Gen Rabbah 46:1 another analogy is given: Rabbi Yudan said, "Just as this fig's only flaw (פסולת) is its stalk, remove it and eliminate the defect (בטל המום). Thus, the Holy Blessed One said to Abraham, 'You have no flaw except your foreskin, remove it and eliminate the defect. Walk before me and be תמים; further in Gen 46:4 we read of another logic for brit milah: Rabbi Levi says it is like a matron to whom the king said, "Pass before me." She passed before him and her face blanched. She thought "what if some flaw is found on me?" The King said to her, "there is no flaw on you except an overgrown nail on your little finger. Remove it and eliminate the defect." Thus said the Holy One to Abraham, "There is no flaw on you except this foreskin. Remove it, and eliminate the defect, and walk before me and be תמים." Apparently speech too can be perfected as Moses and Isaiah both refer to themselves as having "uncircumcised lips" which are purified by divine intervention of fire (a coal in the case of Moshe and seraphim in the case of Isaiah). *Avot de Rabbi Natan* (ARN A 2.5) notes that certain biblical exemplars were born מהול, circumcised, thus in state of bodily perfection, including: Job, Adam, Seth, Noah, Shem, Jacob, Joseph, Moses, Balaam, Samuel, David, Jeremiah, and Zerubavel.

כִּי נֶפֶשׁ הַבָּשָׂר, בַּדָּם הוּא, וַאֲנִי נְתַתִּיו לָכֶם עַל-הַמִּזְבֵּחַ, לְכַפֵּר עַל-נַפְשֹׁתֵיכֶם: כִּי-הַדָּם הוּא, בַּנֶּפֶשׁ יְכַפֵּר.

11 **For the life of the flesh is in the blood**; and I have given it to you upon the altar to make atonement for your souls; for it is the blood that maketh atonement by reason of the life.

In general Plato and the neo-Platonic tradition was also averse to eating blood, however their response was as with Porphyry[24] one of ascetic vegetarianism, while Judaism solved the dilemma by the Kashrut process of salting במלח תמלך (biMalakh timalekh) a process whereby salting meat extracts the blood from the food by a process of osmosis through saturation of the meat

---

[24] The ascetic impulse of third century debates about animal sacrifice, particularly through the prism of Porphyry's *On Abstinence from Killing Animals*, is a vehicle for revealing the coherent understanding of Porphyry on the mechanism by which blood sacrifices fix or embody demonic forces in this world or what Aristotle would call sublunar. As a Platonist Porphyry's asceticism to control animality and low natured lusts, cravings, and desires by abstaining from meat and being a vegetarian, shines through in his argument to control by reason, and not allow the soul to become susceptible to daemons thought to arise from forces of appetite and passion. While Porphyry's advocacy for ascetic vegetarianism, may contradict his own teacher Plotinus' stance, we understand how Porphyry maintains a coherent rational understanding of the origin, nature, and generation of bad daemons by humans consuming blood sacrifices although there is no evidence Porphyry had knowledge of the Biblical prohibition prohibiting the eating of blood "for the life of a creature is in the blood (Lev 3:7; Lev 17:10; Lev 17:4; Deut 12:23; Gen 9:4] which was addressed and ameliorated by the salting process (bimalakh timaleikh) of the Rabbinical system of Kashrut.

with salt, which is later burnt off.[25] Rabbi Yakov Trump in a YU podcast asks, "What is it about salt that makes it indispensable to Jewish life?" and provides an excellent source sheet (mikorot packet) on this topic.[26]   Thus in Judaism the Holy Table of the Temple priesthood is carried over in kashrut, whereby one makes one's dining table into an altar. This transfer from Temple to Rabbinic kashruit became the vehicle for not only the remembrance of the Temple sacrifices, but transfer of holiness and sanctity in the wake of the Hurban not just on the elevated korbanot in which the Kohanim are involved but with regards to the mundane daily necessity in every day life for obtaining nutrients and nutrition via food intake by eating thus elevating the commonplace to something holy and sacroscanct.

Further as a health precaution, In Leviticus 7:26 we read,

וְכָל-דָּם לֹא תֹאכְלוּ, בְּכֹל מוֹשְׁבֹתֵיכֶם, לָעוֹף, וְלַבְּהֵמָה.	**26** And ye shall eat no manner of blood, whether it be of fowl or of beast, in any of your dwellings.

It is know today that blood can transmit deadly infectious diseases. The bible thus contains the first modern public health rules and restrictions against outbreaks of epidemics.

Further consumption of certain types of fat was considered unclean. For example it is commanded

---

וְחֵלֶב נְבֵלָה
וְחֵלֶב טְרֵפָה,
יֵעָשֶׂה
לְכָל-מְלָאכָה;
וְאָכֹל, לֹא
תֹאכְלֻהוּ.

24 And the fat of that which dieth of itself, and the fat of that which is torn of beasts, may be used for any other service; but ye shall in no wise eat of it.

Modern medicine and in particular nephrology recognizes that cleanliness and hygiene can help in part prevent certain types of kidney diseases. [27]

The Rabbinic process of koshering vessels for instance anticipated *avant la lettre*, what has later been shown in infectious disease advances, germ theory, air born microbes, and some kinds of virus transmission, as the process in part involves pouring boiling water or boiling

---

[27] See for instance articles such as: Akar Harun, "**Systemic Consequences of Poor Oral Health in Chronic Kidney Disease Patients** "Published online before print November 2010, doi: 10.2215/CJN.05470610 CJASN January 2011 vol. 6 no. 1 218-226 and J Friberg, "Proteinuria and Kidney Injury among; Workmen exposed to Cadmium and Nickel pust-Preliminary Report".in Journal of Industrial Hygiene and Toxicology 1948 Vol.30 No.1 pp.32-6 ref.17 and Richard Johnson, "Hypothesis: dysregulation of immunologic balance resulting from hygiene and socioeconomic factors may influence the epidemiology and cause of glomerulonephritis worldwide" in American Journal of Kidney Diseases September 2003 Volume 42, Issue 3, Pages 575–581; See MC Freeman in **Systematic review: hygiene and health: systematic review of handwashing practices worldwide and update of health effects**; MG Lankford in **Influence of role models and hospital design on the hand hygiene of health-care workers**; JE Park in **Textbook of preventive and social medicine: a treatise on community health**; J Bartram in **Hygiene, sanitation, and water: forgotten foundations of health**; The World Health Organization guidelines on hand hygiene in health care and their consensus recommendations; London School of Hygiene and Tropical Medicine; PDR Johnson in **Efficacy of an alcohol/chlorhexidine hand hygiene program in a hospital with high rates of nosocomial methicillin-resistant Staphylococcus aureus (MRSA)**; N Tomes in Bulletin of the History of Medicine, **The private side of public health: sanitary science, domestic hygiene, and the germ theory, 1870-1900**; D Pittet in **Hand hygiene among physicians: performance, beliefs, and perceptions**; V Curtis in **Domestic hygiene and diarrhoea–pinpointing the problem**; AM Grant and DM Hoffman in **It's not all about me: motivating hand hygiene among health care professionals by focusing on patients**; A Pruss-Ustam in **Burden of disease from inadequate water, sanitation and hygiene in low–and middle–income settings: a retrospective analysis of data from 145 countries**; JD Siegel 2007 guideline for isolation precautions: preventing transmission of infectious agents in health care settings; etc

vessels such as dishes in hot water. Thus this rabbinic process anticipates major break throughs in epidemic investigations and the key work of Louis Pasteur in areas such as Pasteurization in 19th century France. The emphasis on hygiene and cleanliness in the Bible we thus see are insights much *avant la lettre* in subsequent discoveries in medicine and science.[28]

Kidneys as Seat of Emotions, Conscience, Desire, Thought, Affections, and Sensation[29]

In the Bible the kidneys are related to the seat of sensation and lust. According to Mishlei (23:16) the kidneys rejoice when the lips speak right things: וְתַעְלֹזְנָה כִלְיוֹתָי-- בְּדַבֵּר שְׂפָתֶיךָ, מֵישָׁרִים Likewise kidneys are the site of faithfulness when we hear in Isaiah 11:5

וְהָיָה צֶדֶק, אֵזוֹר מָתְנָיו; וְהָאֱמוּנָה, אֵזוֹר חֲלָצָיו.	**5** And righteousness shall be the girdle of his loins, and faithfulness the girdle of his reins

Kidneys can also express concern or grief such as when we are taught in Psalms 73:21

כִּי, יִתְחַמֵּץ לְבָבִי; וְכִלְיוֹתַי, אֶשְׁתּוֹנָן.	**21** For my heart was in a ferment, and I was pricked in my reins

---

[28] See The Bible and Modern Medicine, London, The Paternoster Press, 1955

[29] See Levin, SS, Adam's Rib: Essays on Biblical Medicine, Los Altos, Geron-X, Inc 1970

According to the author of Iyov (19:27), Job's kidneys withered within him because of his yearning: ,אֲשֶׁר אֲנִי .אֶחֱזֶה-לִּי--וְעֵינַי רָאוּ וְלֹא-זָר: כָּלוּ כִלְיֹתַי בְּחֵקִי Job feels what nobody else can detect, that his kidneys (the innermost organs) are demolished and therefore he sees no hope of recovery because "counsel is no more." Later in Iyov (38:36) it is said that the L-rd places wisdom in the kidneys: מִי-שָׁת, בַּטֻּחוֹת חָכְמָה; אוֹ מִי-נָתַן לַשֶּׂכְוִי בִינָה In the prophet Jeremiah (11:20) we learn that the L-rd tests the heart and kidneys: וַיהוָה צְבָאוֹת שֹׁפֵט צֶדֶק, בֹּחֵן כְּלָיוֹת וָלֵב; אֶרְאֶה נִקְמָתְךָ מֵהֶם, כִּי אֵלֶיךָ גִּלִּיתִי אֶת-רִיבִי A physician may test the pulse from the heart, and the urine from the kidneys, in order to indirectly conclude things about the health of an individual's heart and kidneys, but only the L-rd however, who knows the innermost wisdom of the human body and all things tests the heart and kidneys directly, by just knowing the health of the person without interpreting the physiological signs of the blood and urine. The Biblical phrase to "test the heart and kidneys" presupposes on the part of the rabbis the correct medical observation of the inter relationship of the two organs in the field of nephrology.

The kidneys are also evoked in the Bible as the most innermost, hidden, and mysterious of organs with regards to embryology.[30] In Psalm 139:16 we read:

---

[30] See Kottek, Samuel, "Embryology in Bible and Talmud", J Hist of Biology 14, (1981), p. 299-315

טז גָּלְמִי, רָאוּ עֵינֶיךָ, וְעַל-סִפְרְךָ, כֻּלָּם יִכָּתֵבוּ: יָמִים יֻצָּרוּ; וְלֹא (וְלוֹ) אֶחָד בָּהֶם.

16 Thine eyes did see mine unformed substance, and in Thy book they were all written-- even the days that were fashioned, when as yet there was none of them.

The Psalmist then extols the all knowing G-d whose thought is not like human thought but rather all knowing: G-d וְלִי--מַה-יָּקְרוּ רֵעֶיךָ אֵל; מֶה עָצְמוּ, רָאשֵׁיהֶם even knows what man will see before speaking: כִּי אֵין מִלָּה, בִּלְשׁוֹנִי; הֵן ד', יָדַעְתָּ כֻלָּהּ Then the Psalmist notes that G-d's greatest wisdom process in embryological development is the formation of the kidneys:

כִּי-אַתָּה, קָנִיתָ כִלְיֹתָי; תְּסֻכֵּנִי, בְּבֶטֶן אִמִּי.

13 For Thou hast made my reins; Thou hast knit me together in my mother's womb.

The Psalmist proclaims this formation of the kidneys "wonderous and marevelous:

אוֹדְךָ-- עַל כִּי נוֹרָאוֹת, נִפְלֵיתִי: נִפְלָאִים מַעֲשֶׂיךָ; וְנַפְשִׁי, יֹדַעַת מְאֹד.

14 I will give thanks unto Thee, for I am fearfully and wonderfully made; wonderful are Thy works; and that my soul knoweth right well.

The creation of the kidneys is singled out, no other organ being referred to in this sequence of G-d's wonderous acts. Why are the kidney's singled out as the epitome of God's wisdom in forming? Rabbi Abraham ibn Ezra gives three reasons, the primary being that the kidneys are the "most remote innermost organs placed in a secret abode.[31]

The rabbis called urine *sheten* although the usual term is *meme raglayim* meaning "water of the feet." The rabbis were aware of knowledge imparted by the turbity or consistency of the urine. For instance Rabbi Shesheth is said to observe the physiology of urine in horses and camels as not thick. However he notes that the water of a donkey is thick and resembles milk. Based on the principle "that which goes out from the unclean is unclean" (i.e donkeys are not kosher) the question is raised in the gemarah (Berachoth 7b) if the thick urine of an ass may be used in medications?

The kidneys are also considered the site of affections as in expressing joy where we read in Mishlei 23:16

טו בְּנִי, אִם-חָכַם לִבֶּךָ-- יִשְׂמַח לִבִּי גַם-אָנִי.	**15** My son, if thy heart be wise, my heart will be glad, even mine;
טז וְתַעְלֹזְנָה כִלְיוֹתָי-- בְּדַבֵּר שְׂפָתֶיךָ, מֵישָׁרִים.	**16** Yea, my reins will rejoice, when thy lips speak right things.

---

[31] Ibn Ezra's other two reasons are (1) They are related to the heart being as it were its counterpart in the lower part of the body. And (2) They are also the seat of understanding and of feeling, perhaps even of moral and ethical consciousness according to Ibn Ezra.

The heart and he kidneys are thus associated with both the seat of joy and felicity in this pusek of *mishlei* related to ethical conduct (*darkheim noam*) and rightful speaking (*loshon naki*).

In Jeremiah it further is asserted (12:2) that the L-rd is near to the mouth of the wicked and far from the kidneys: קָרוֹב אַתָּה בְּפִיהֶם, וְרָחוֹק מִכִּלְיוֹתֵיהֶם That is to say the hypocrites, who God hates, merely pay lip service to the L-rd but do not feel fear of God's ability to see into the inward parts i.e. the kidneys considered the most inward of all organs. When the *navi* Jeremiah was threatened by his enemies he exclaimed "O Lord of Hosts that does judge righteously who does try the kidneys and the heart (*bohen kelayot va-lev*) let me see thy vengeance on them (my enemies)."[32]

In Chullin 55a it is disputed if the "white of the kidney" is included in the Biblical concept of forbidden tallow The rabbis with their careful inspection slaughtered animals according to Kashrut, knew the kidney is covered by a double membrane. The outer membrane, the fat capsule, is prohibited fat. The inner membrane, the *capsula fibrosa* contains abundant fibres. According to Leviticus 3:4 the fat which is on the kidneys which must be offered in the Temple lies outside both membranes:

וְהִקְרִיב מִזֶּבַח הַשְּׁלָמִים, אִשֶּׁה לַד'—אֶת-הַחֵלֶב, הַמְכַסֶּה
אֶת-הַקֶּרֶב, וְאֵת כָּל-הַחֵלֶב, אֲשֶׁר עַל-הַקֶּרֶב.
וְאֵת, שְׁתֵּי הַכְּלָיֹת, וְאֶת-הַחֵלֶב אֲשֶׁר עֲלֵהֶן, אֲשֶׁר עַל-הַכְּסָלִים;
וְאֶת-הַיֹּתֶרֶת, עַל-הַכָּבֵד, עַל-הַכְּלָיוֹת, יְסִירֶנָּה.
וְהִקְטִירוּ אֹתוֹ בְנֵי-אַהֲרֹן, הַמִּזְבֵּחָה, עַל-הָעֹלָה, אֲשֶׁר
עַל-הָעֵצִים אֲשֶׁר עַל-הָאֵשׁ--אִשֵּׁה רֵיחַ נִיחֹחַ, לַד'

---

[32] This image of trying the kidneys appears in Psalms 7:10 and Psalms 26:2

[and he shall present of the sacrifice of peace-offerings an offering made by fire unto the LORD: the fat that covereth the inwards, and all the fat that is upon the inwards,/ and the two kidneys, and the fat that is on them, which is by the loins, and the lobe above the liver, which he shall take away hard by the kidneys./ And Aaron's sons shall make it smoke on the altar upon the burnt-offering, which is upon the wood that is on the fire; it is an offering made by fire, of a sweet savour unto the LORD.]

In Becharoth 39a Rabbi Chiya states that an animal can have one, or even three kidneys, but this is an unusual congenital basis. The rabbis of course know that is normal to have two kidneys. Rabbi Yochanan disputes the possibility of an animal being born with one kidney, what is called teratologic renal anomalies, which is not normal, or the usual course in envisioning the symmetry of two eyes, two ears, two feet, two hands, two kidneys etc. He thus excluded the medical rare phenomena of the solitary kidney or accessory kidney. The existence of an animal born with three kidneys is cited in Bekhorot 39a.

Hazal ruled that an animal which has lost both kidneys is fit for food (kasher).[33] See Hullin 3:2

משנה מסכת חולין פרק ג
ואלו כשרות בבהמה ניקבה הגרגרת או שנסדקה עד כמה
תחסר רבן שמעון בן גמליאל אומר עד כאיסר האיטלקי
נפחתה הגלגלת ולא ניקב קרום של מוח ניקב הלב ולא לבית
חללו נשברה השדרה ולא נפסק החוט שלה ניטלה הכבד
ונשתייר הימנה כזית המסס ובית הכוסות שניקבו זה לתוך

---

[33] Kottek suggests that this ruling may be influenced by Aristotle who writes, "The kidneys when they are extant are suited to serve in the execretion of the fluid which collects in the bladder. (De Part Anim. II, 7, 670b23-26. Kottek further notes that for Pliny, "all viviparous quadrupeds have kidneys" (Nat. Hist. XI: 81).

זה ניטל הטחול ניטלו הכליות ניטל לחי התחתון ניטל האם
שלה וחרותה בידי שמים הגלודה רבי מאיר מכשיר וחכמים
פוסלין:

However the Talmud considers even one diseased kidney to be dangerous to render the animal unfit (taref).[34] According to Hazal a partially damaged kidney does not regenerate (Hullin 128b).

In Berachoth 61a the kidneys are viewed as the advisors of the heart. According to Genesis Rabbah 61:1 since Abraham could not learn wisdom from his father and since he had no teacher, his kidneys played a role of teacher. Avraham's ability to develop and recognize the truth of ethical monotheism regarding G-d came from within, specifically identified with the advice of his kidneys.[35]

Avraham Who Learned Advice From His Kidneys
Ethical Monotheism

Genesis Rabbah 61:1 is the source of an enigmatic remark that tells that Avraham was taught the law by his kidneys and then developed the recognition of God from within. Berkhot 61a reads:

> The kidneys give advice (kelayot yo'azot),the heart comprehends (mevin), the tongue articulated

---

[34] Hullin 25a & 25b.;

[35] [see Kottek, Samuel S. "The Kidneys give advice: Some thoughts on nephrology in the Talmud and Midrash" in Koroth 10 (1933-1994), 44-53, 1993]

(literally cuts), and the mouth concludes (gomer).[36]

Thus the kidneys are the counsellors of the heart. In Leviticus Rabba 4:4 we see a similar idea that the kidneys are the counselors of the soul:

> Ten things minister to the soul; the oesophagus for food, the trachea for the voice, the liver for anger, the lung for liquids, the gullet for grinding, the spleen for laughing, the stomach for sleeping, the gall for lust (literally jealousy*), the kidneys for thinking (mehashevot),* the heart finishes off (or completes, brings to perfection, or organizes the whole physiological process, Hebrew gomer), and the soul stands above all these organs

This idea of the kidney as the site of advice and counsel is found in Psalms 16:7 where we read:

אֲבָרֵךְ—אֶת-ד',	**7** I will bless the LORD, who
אֲשֶׁר יְעָצָנִי;	hath given me counsel; yea, in
אַף-לֵילוֹת, יִסְּרוּנִי	the night seasons my reins
כִלְיוֹתָי.	instruct me (yisserun)

---

[36] See also: Hullin 11a, Shabbat 33b, Koheleth Rabbati 7:36; Avot de Rabbi Nathan 31:3; Full text is: The oesophagus takes in. all kinds of edibles, the trachea (qaneh) brings forth the voice, the lungs imbibe all kinds of liquors, the liver causes anger, the bile instils in it one drop and thus calms it down (calms liver), the spleen causes laughter, the gullet grinds, the stomach causes sleep, the noses wakes him up...." קהלת
רבה (וילנא) פרשה ז:

מעשרה שליטים שמשמשין את הנפש, ואלו הן, הושט למזון, קנה לקול,
כבד לחמה, מרה לקנאה, הריאה מששתן, המסס לטחון, טחול לשחוק כליות
יועצות, לב מבין, לשון גומר.

The kidneys are hidden in mystery as they are concealed in the inner parts. They metaphorically represent the innermost loci if thought and desire, hardly accessible or in the direct consciousness of man and plane sight, but readily seen and tested by the L-rd. It is from this mysterium that Avraham learned of ethical monotheism. Genesis 26:5 states that Avraham Avinu knew and practiced all the ordinances of the Torah which were later revealed to Moshe Rabbenu centuries later.

If Sinaitic revelation was centuries later in Shemot, how did Avraham learn Torah? His father was said to own an idol shop in Haran and Ur so it was not from Terah. According to Rabbi Shimon, the L-rd inspired Abraham's two kidneys, which became his teachers[37]

---

[37] Another opinion is that Avraham, Yitchak, and Yakov learned Torah in the yeshivah of Shem (Noah's son) and Ever (Shem's son); See Midrash Rabbah בראשית רבה (וילנא) פרשת נח פרשה לז Gen. 37:10;

ולשם יולד גם הוא אבי כל בני עבר וגו', אין אנו יודעין אם שם הוא הגדול אם יפת הוא הגדול, מן מה דכתיב אלה תולדות שם בן מאת שנה ויולד את ארפכשד שנתים אחר המבול הוי יפת הוא הגדול, ולעבר יולד שני בנים שם האחד פלג כי בימיו נפלגה הארץ, רבי יוסי ורשב"ג רבי יוסי אומר הראשונים ע"י שהיו מכירים את יחוסיהם היו מוציאין שמן לשם המאורע, אבל אנו שאין אנו מכירים את יחוסינו, אנו מוציאין לשם אבותינו, רשב"ג אומר הראשונים על ידי שהיו משתמשין ברוח הקודש, היו מוציאין לשם המאורע, אבל אנו שאין אנו משתמשין ברוח הקודש אנו מוציאין לשם אבותינו, א"ר יוסי בן חלפתא נביא גדול היה עבר שהוציא לשם המאורע הה"ד ולעבר יולד שני בנים וגו', למה נקרא שמו יקטן, שהיה מקטין את עצמו ואת עסקיו, ומה זכה, זכה להעמיד י"ג משפחות, ומה אם הקטן שהוא מקטין עסקיו כך, גדול שהוא מקטין את עסקיו על אחת כמה וכמה, ודכוותה (בראשית מח) וישלח ישראל את ימינו וישת על ראש אפרים והוא הצעיר, אמר רבי הונא וכי מן התולדות אין אנו יודעין שהוא הצעיר, אלא שהיה מצעיר את עסקיו, ומה זכה, זכה לבכורה, ומה אם הצעיר על ידי שהיה מצעיר את עסקיו זכה לבכורה, גדול שהוא מצעיר את עסקיו על אחת כמה וכמה See also Kuzari I:95.

and infused in him Torah and wisdom (*torah ve-hokmah*).[38] We thus learn from Midrash Rabba Gen. 61:1

בראשית רבה (וילנא) פרשת חיי שרה פרשה סא
כי אם בתורת ה' חפצו, כי ידעתיו למען אשר יצוה, ובתורתו
יהגה אר"ש אב לא למדו ורב לא היה לו, ומהיכן למד את
התורה, אלא זימן לו הקב"ה שתי כליותיו כמין שני רבנים
והיו נובעות ומלמדות אותו תורה וחכמה, הה"ד (תהלים טז)
אברך את ה' אשר יעצני אף לילות יסרוני כליותי,
(שם /תהלים/ א) והיה כעץ שתול ששתלו הקב"ה בארץ
ישראל, אשר פריו יתן בעתו זה ישמעאל ועלהו לא יבול זה
יצחק, וכל אשר יעשה יצליח אלו בני קטורה שנאמר ויוסף
אברהם ויקח אשה.

---

[38] See Yoma 28b; Mishnah Kidushin 4:14 משנה מסכת קידושין
פרק ד

משנה יד

[*] ר' יהודה אומר לא ירעה רווק בהמה ולא ישנו שני רווקים בטלית אחת
וחכמים מתירין כל שעסקו עם הנשים לא יתייחד עם הנשים ולא ילמד אדם
את בנו אומנות בין הנשים רבי מאיר אומר לעולם ילמד אדם את בנו אומנות
נקיה וקלה ויתפלל למי שהעושר והנכסים שלו שאין אומנות שאין בה עניות
ועשירות שלא עניות מן האומנות ולא עשירות מן האומנות אלא הכל לפי
זכותו רבי שמעון בן אלעזר אומר ראית מימיך חיה ועוף שיש להם אומנות
והן מתפרנסין שלא בצער והלא לא נבראו אלא לשמשני ואני נבראתי לשמש
את קוני איני דין שאתפרנס שלא בצער אלא שהרעותי מעשי וקפחתי את
פרנסתי אבא גוריין איש צדיין אומר משום אבא גוריא לא ילמד אדם את בנו
חמר גמל ספן רועה וחנוני שאומנתן אומנות לסטים רבי יהודה אומר
משמו החמרין רובן רשעים והגמלין רובן כשרים הספנין רובן חסידים טוב
שברופאים לגיהנם והכשר שבטבחים שותפו של עמלק רבי נהוראי אומר
מניח אני כל אומנות שבעולם ואיני מלמד את בני אלא תורה שאדם אוכל
משכרה בעולם הזה וקרן קיימת לעולם הבא ושאר כל אומנות אינן כן
כשאדם בא לידי חולי או לידי זקנה או לידי יסורין ואינו יכול לעסוק
במלאכתו הרי הוא מת ברעב אבל התורה אינה כן אלא משמרתו מכל רע
בנערותו ונותנת לו אחרית ותקוה בזקנותו בנערותו מה הוא אומר (ישעיה מ')
וקוי ה' יחליפו כח בזקנותו מהו אומר (תהלים צ"ב) עוד ינובון בשיבה וכן
הוא אומר באברהם אבינו עליו השלום (בראשית כ"ד) ואברהם זקן וה' ברך
את אברהם בכל מצינו שעשה אברהם אבינו את כל התורה כולה עד שלא
נתנה שנאמר (שם /בראשית/ כ"ו) עקב אשר שמע אברהם בקולי וישמור
משמרתי מצותי חקותי ותורותי:
סליקא לה מסכת קדושין וסדר נשים בסייעתא דשמיא

Another tradition teaches, also ascribed to Rabbi Shimon bar Yohai (Rashbi), is that Abraham's two kidneys functioned like two flasks of water which introduced the Torah into him. We should recall the agadata of Rabbi Akiva who proclaimed that if a stream could make a dent in a stone in the riverbed, then words of Torah could seep into his soul before he started learning Torah. Yet Rabbi Akiva when he reaches the throne of Hashem in the account of the *arba sheniknasu biPardes* in Hagigah 12b-14b says, "*Al tamru mayim, mayim.*"[39] Hazal associate water with Torah. For example in Isaiah 12:2-3 which is incorporated into Havdalah we read:

הִנֵּה אֵל יְשׁוּעָתִי אֶבְטַח,	2 Behold, God is my salvation; I
וְלֹא אֶפְחָד: כִּי-עָזִּי	will trust, and will not be afraid;
וְזִמְרָת יָהּ ד', וַיְהִי-לִי	for GOD the LORD is my strength
לִישׁוּעָה.	and song; and He is become my
	salvation.'

---

[39] The simple peshat noted by Josephus is that Rabbi Akiva who had seen before the Hurban the Beit HaMikdash, had witnessed the beautiful pure blue marble. When the sun was up and the sunlight bounced off the gold dome of the Temple the blue painted marble, appeared as shimmering waters of the Mediterranean sea. This reminds one of the gemarah in Hullin that the blue threads remind one of the blue waters of the Mediterranean sea which remind one of the rakiah which remind one of the throne of G-d which is also the color of the luchot. Thus Rabbi Akiva who entered and exited in peace unlike the other 3 who ventured into the Pardes may be saying do not be fooled by the appearance of the light on the pure blue marble that appears as shimmering waters. A messianic King will arise who judges not "by the hearing of the ears" (motzi shem rah) or the "seeing of the eyes" but by truth, justice, and fairness. The waters taken on deeper significance referencing the waters that are above the heavens (*hamayim ma-al ha-shamayim*) and the waters below the heavens (hamayim me-*tachat ha-shamayim*) which in turn may refer to what sifrei Kabbalah refer to as the *mayim elyonim* and the *mayim tachtonim*.

וּשְׁאַבְתֶּם-מַיִם,   ג   **3** Therefore with joy shall ye draw
בְּשָׂשׂוֹן, מִמַּעַיְנֵי,   water out of the wells of salvation
הַיְשׁוּעָה.

Likewise in Samuel II 22:18 Dovid HaMelekh proclaims on the seventh day of Pesah in the Haftorah:

{ס}   יִשְׁלַח מִמָּרוֹם, יִקָּחֵנִי;   **17** He sent from on high, He
יַמְשֵׁנִי, מִמַּיִם רַבִּים. {ר}   took me; He drew me out of
many waters

Water is associated with the blessing of rain as on Sukkot in the tefilat geshem.[40] Urine was referred to as water

---

[40] The prayer reads: Af-Bri is designated as the name of the angel of rain to thicken and to form clouds, to empty them, and to cause rain.. Water with which to crown the valley's vegetation- may it not be withheld because of our unredeemed debt. In the memory of the faithful Patriarchs protect the ones who pray for rain... May He obligate the Angel Af-Bri to give us portions of the segregated rain, to soften the wasteland's face when it is dry as a rock. With water you symbolized Your might in Scripture, to soothe with its drops those in whom was blown a soul to keep alive the ones who recall the strength of the rain... Remember the patriarch Avraham who was drawn behind You like water. You blessed him like a tree replanted alongside streams of water. You shielded him you rescued him from fire and from water. You tested him when he sowed upon all waters.... Remember Isaac born with the tidings of Let some water be brought. You told his father to offer him- to spill his blood like water. He too was scrupulous to pour his heart like water. He dug and discovered wells of water..... Remember Yakov who carried his staff and crossed the Jordan's water. He dedicated his heart and rolled away a stone off the mouth of a well of water. As when he wrestled by an angel composed of fire and water. Therefore You pledged to remain with him through fire and water.... The prayer goes on to associate water with Moses, Aaron and the twelve trives. This prayer for rain is also related to the prayer for dew on Pesah, as dew is associated with the Dews of resurrection.

from between the feet (*mei raglayim*).[41] Nonetheless pure water was a symbol of learning. Thus in Hagigah 3a we learn "we are your disciples and we are drinking your waters (i.e. Torah), as two of his pupils said to Rabbi Yehoshua. The kidneys function making water even at night unseen to man. Thus "my kidneys admonish me during the night."

Avraham is said to have brought many individuals under the wings of the *Shekhinah* of the "souls that Avraham made" by imparting a belief and understanding, as far as the limits of human understanding can grasp, of the oneness and uniqueness of G-d. Philosophers after Avraham, including Rav Saadia Gaon in *Sefer Emunot Ve-Deot*, Rav Bachya ibn Pakudah in *Hovoot LeVavot*, Rabbi Yehudah HaLevy in the *Kuzari*, Maimonides in the *Moreh HaNevukhim*, and others, gave rational proofs for the existence and uniqueness of Hashem. Avraham came to an understanding of monotheism, and how this belief and position leads one to naturally conclude that G-d created the world, *yesh mi-ayin* (creation ex nihilo) rather than other positions in philosophy that the world is eternal (Aristotle's position), or creation *de novo* (Plato's position). If we believe in creation *ex nihilo* (*yesh mi-ayin*)

---

[41] It was considered unbecoming to urinate in or near the Jersualem Temple. Berakhot 40a considered it unbecoming to have one's feet soiled by drops of urine. Thus pilgrims to the Temple would immerse (tevel) in a mikvah before entering the Temple's staircase. See b. Yoma 29a, Mishnah, Makhshirim 6:5.

it follows logically that creationism indicates a unique, perfect, self-sufficient Creator.[42]

The attempt to "prove" ethical monotheism is thus a cognizant seeking for a divine entity with regard to the fact that it is unique and self-sufficient and perfect and with regard to its Being qua being, as it is (*in seinem Dass-und Sosein*). The attempt for "proof" is thus encapsulated in the Psalmists proclamation, "*Do not hide Your presence from me*" (Ps. 27:9).

As Wittgenstein, a philosophic mathematician noted, a proposition [i.e. G-d exists (Hu Kayam)] "that has sense states something" [*Der sinnvolle Satz sagt etwas aus*], which is shown by its proof (*Beweis*) to be so.

---

[42] While the attempts to prove G-d's existence are many in the course of philosophy, a number of those proofs from medieval Jewish philosophers are classified under some the following categories: (1) proof from motions, (2) proof from intelligent design, (3) ontological proof, (4) efficient cause proof, or proof from causality, (4) argument of necessary Being who is perfect and self-sufficient, (5) argument from gradation, (6) argument from moral conscience, (7) from reliable tradition, (8) credo absurdum ist, (9), universal consent. Medieval Jewish theologians like Rav Sadia Gaon, Rav Bachya, Rav Yehudah HaLevy, and Maimonides who all offer "proofs" for the existence of a unique monotheistic Deity, understand these "proofs" as drawing on philosophical method as a most important ancilla theologiae. The medieval Jewish philosophers who offer demonstrations of "proofs" for a unique monotheistic Deity understand that "proof" is a kind of ontological seeking (Suchen) for every seeking for or questing for human understanding is guided beforehand by that which is sought i.e. G-d's essence. Yet Maimonides shows that G-d's essence cannot be known in the sense we cannot put G-d in a box i.e G-d's essence cannot be "limited", "framed", or put in a human conceptual boundry i.e. G-d is transcendent. So what do the Medieval Jewish philosophers attempting to demonstrate the existence of One Unique Deity understand as constituting their demonstration before the "tribunal of reason" of the truth claims of revelation?

Wittgenstein's *Tractatus Logico-Philosophicus*, employs the method of Euclidean gemotric proof, to demonstrate in 7 carefully epistemologically organized propositions, that "the world is all that is the case" however "*Wovon mann nicht sprechen kann daruber muss mann schweigen)*- a secular form in some sense of the the ontological proof for G-d's unique existence. However where the medieval Jewish proofs for G-d's existence, uniqueness, perfection, self-sufficiency, not being finite, not being corporeal, etc. differ from the modern Wittgenstinain "system building" post-Hegel, making (poesis), or constructing, is clear in that the medieval philosophers reject substitution of something else for G-d, even a scientific system. All this Avraham learned from his kidneys the Midrash states. The medieval philosophers faithfully reject attempts to make G-d's presence controllable by human *techne*. That is to say as religiously grounded philosophers who accept the truth claims of revelation, and know how to demonstrate their truth before the tribunal of reason, the medieval religious Jewish philosophers understand the verse, "*Behold the very heavens do not contain You*" (I Kgs. 8:27) for G-d in geometic terms is a "circle whose circumference is infinite" i.e. not finite, in the *loshon of Kabbalah- ayn sof.* The uniqueness of the medieval Jewish philosophers' apprehension of G-d via revelation is encapsulated in the verse, "*Has a people ever heard the voice of G-d speaking from the midst of fire as you have heard and lived* (Deut. 4:33). A difference between medieval religious proofs for the existence of G-d and the modern Wittgenstinian proofs for the existence of all that is in nature, scientifically mapped, is that for the medievals "man and his humanly constructed proofs are not the measure of all things". The medieval religious sensibility looks on man's "constructed technological inventions i.e. proofs that follow the laws of logic and reason" as caused by G-d for the sake of the covenant. That is to say the medieval Jewish philosophic proofs for a monotheistic Deity are always conscious that, "*And you shall remember the L-rd your G-d, that it is He who gives you strength to make wealth in order to uphold His covenant"* (Deut. 8:18). Thus for the medievals versus the moderns, the Torah is not viewed as the means to the end of technolgocial success with constructing understandings of nature. Rather the world is looked upon as the means for man to observe Torah as Avraham understood Thus the halakhocentrism of medieval Jewish thought.

The ontological proof which posits that "G-d is the thought beyond which thought cannot proceed" moves from the concept of a Supreme Perfect Being (*ens realissimum*) to absolute existence in relation to contingent existence (see Plato[43] and Rorty on contingency of opinions held by the many which are false), while the cosmological argument (G-d as *First Cause (siva Rishona)* who put in motion the heavenly bodies in their orbits) moves from the experience of the contingent existence of the world (*a contingentia mundi*) to the concept of a Supreme Perfect Being and His absolute existence. Anselm much later than medieval Jewish philosophers like Rav Sadia Gaon, Rav Bachya, and Maimonides before him, put it this way: "we believe that You are a Being beyond which nothing greater can be conceived (*aliquid quo maius nihil cogitari non potest; see Proslogion,* ch.2). It goes without saying that "textbook" identification of William Paley as the founder of the ontological proof is also much *apres la lettre*.

Science learns from observation, method and testing. Experientially i.e. phenomenologically, respect for the

---

[43] For Plato, the body is ephemeral but the soul immortal and after death if worthy enters the true realm of the forms. However Plato's view of the body is also complex. See Jouboud C, Le Corps Humain dans la philosophie Platonicienne, Etude a partir du Timee, Paris: Librarie Philosophique J Vrin, 1991

structure of nature (the laws of nature i.e. law of gravity, entropy, thermodynamics, Einsteinian relativity theory, and string theory and unified field theory today) reminds us that one cannot reduce G-d's presence to human limited experience of it. *"Then the L-rd answered Job out of the whirlwind, saying... I will question you and you may inform Me. Where were you when I laid the foundations of the earth? Tell me if you have any understanding* (Iyov 38:1,3). *Yesh mi-ayin* or creation ex nihilo posits a Supreme Orderer who is immanent in His creation (i.e. establishes laws of nature which scientists seek out to discover G-d's hidden ordering structures as Hume remarks "nature loves to hide"), yet a Creator *ex nihilo* transcends His world which is a theological paradox- i.e. *"Thus says the L-rd: the heaven is My throne and the earth My footstool for all of these things My hand has made and all of these things have come to be...* (Isa. 66:1-2). The medieval Jewish philosophers understand however that "human making" is not "divine Creative making" as the verb *"bara"* is specific to G-d's creative action. Thus the *teological argument* sees G-d's presence though the "value" of the world, and the cosmological argument sees G-d's presence through the structure/ divine order established in the nature of the world etc. The existence of miracles as deriving uniquely from G-d thus is revealed whether we are with Maimonides that the messianic era is a political state of affairs where the Jews will not be persecuted as laid out in *sefer Shoftim of the mishneh Torah,* or as Rabbi Don Isaac Abarbanel holds that the messiah will indeed perform miracles via the workings of the *ruach hakodesh*.[44] Further whether we understand miracle as a breaking of the laws that G-d established in nature, or G-d's manipulating of those laws to effect a change in the usual order of nature (the sun stood still for Joshua) is moot. Medieval debates continue if the parting of the Read Sea, a divine miracle as factum, is constituted by the "timing" of the parting of

---

[44] Rambam and Abarbanel differ over positions regarding Jewish philosophic views on the ideas of the messianism, and related areas such as *yamim ahronim, ikvot ha-mashiah, afterlife, geulah, tihiyat ha-maytim, olam ha-ba, Gan Eden.* Two defining messianic approaches and the schematic process of future redemption. Maimonides' naturalistic model emphasizes that nature will not undergo a fundamental change [עבע השתנות] and diverts focus to the individual redemption of the philosophic soul by achieving perfection (shelamuth) of the intellect through divine noetic communion. Saadia and Ramban supported differing forms of apocalyptic messianism based on supernatural miracles, wonders (nifla'ot), and changes in nature. poles of naturalism and apocalyptic messianism that provide the measurement for classifying various messianic outlooks that emerged in Medieval Jewish rationalism. One pole in defining the messianic schema is characteristic of Maimonideans is understanding redemption as restoration to the golden age of King David and Solomon when the Temple stands. Rambam gives objective rational criteria for this era: no more war (after Gog and Magog), no more famine, re-existence of the Sanhedrin, reinstitution of laws of *shemitah, yovel,* blessings abundant. Rambam suggests that TB Shabbat 30b & Ketuboth 111b which figuratively speaks of miracles that Eretz Yisrael will produce cakes ready baked and garments of fine silk, just denotes the abundance and ease of blessings. For Rambam the one preoccupation of world will be to know Hashem so that the knowledge of Hashem will be as widespread as waters in the sea. Rambam emphasizes the criteria by which humans may perfect their intellect in communion with eternal truths to cognize the divine intelligible order of the cosmos, and G-d's attributes (not a body, not finite, not ignorant, etc), and uncovering secrets in the Torah reconciled in harmony with science. The Rambam thus interprets anthropomorphisms philosophically (i.e. *BiTzelem Elokim* means endowment with the *sekel ha-poel*) and midrashim such as the feast of leviathan (TB Berkhot 34a, TB Sanhedrin 99a) are taken figuratively since there is nothing physical in *olam ha-bah* but the righteous sit with crowns on their heads basking in the *ziv shekhinah* (TB Berakhot 17a). Rambam follows the position of Shmuel (TB Berakhot 34b & Sanhedrin 91b) where Shmuel posits the sole difference between the world and *biyamei ha-machiah* is delivery from bondage to foreign powers, which becomes the bastion of messianic naturalism. Thus the Rambam interprets "a wolf will dwell with the kid" (Isa 5:6) as a mushal whereby the Jews are the lambs and the wolves the persecuting nations (Jer.5:6).
The other pole on the spectrum of the messianic model in Rabbinic thought is supernatural apocalypticism represented by the Ramban and Abarbanel. This involves the end of the present world through the collapse of history (not as described *après la lettre* by Hegel) and its predetermined onset which runs according to esoteric calculations, detailing for instance *shemitah ha-olamot,* like clockwork hidden in the Hebrew calendar. Accompanying the dramatic end will be a series of catastrophic events involving the extinction of one part of humanity and destruction of the cosmos (3). A new order will replace the present natural world order. Instincts will be changed [what Tirosh-Samuelson calls transhumanism] and people will live forever. A new reality will emerge on the ruins of the present order. The apocalypticists often take *aggadah* literally and prophecies *verbatim,* such as "new heavens and a new earth" (Isa 65:17; 66:22). Thus paradise and resurrection of the dead, the day of the L-rd are actual places and events. The thrust of apocalypticism is public and does not emphasize, Maimonidean individual redemption of the intellect, for apocalyptics subsume the individual into cosmic and national events.

the sea- that it parted just when the children of Israel needed it to part, or whether its parting was a function of G-d drawing on the laws of nature (i.e. strong winds?) which He set in place to govern the natural world etc.

The important point being that Jewish philosophers have attempted to demonstrate ethical monotheism in the course of Jewish history by philosophic proofs, understanding at the same time that G-d's essence cannot be known and human beings, in their limited cognitive capacity will never be able to "frame-limit-or put a boundry" on Hashem's infinite power. Avraham long knew this before medieval philosophy as when he smashed his father's idols knowing that God's transcendence cannot be put in a frame, limit, or box. Thus part of what *Avraham Avinu* perceived, as the early teacher of ethical monotheism, is that G-d's authority is not a function of "capriciousness" for G-d is the ulitmate Judge who is ultimately Just. *Tzedek tzedek tirdof.* Thus Avraham can ask, "*Shall the Judge of the whole earth not do justice?*" (Gen. 18:25). No proof of G-d's existence, no matter how divinely inspired or inventive, will perhaps never do justice to that which it seeks to demonstrate by the nature of the fact that G-d's transcendent omniscience, incorporeality, and infinity can not be "controlled" by human beings. If anyone possesses delusions of grandeur that they can control G-d in any way they are idolators. For it was Avraham who showed that attempts to "feed an idol", "appease an idol", or "bribe an idol", or "worship an idol of stone and wood" in any way constitutes a violation of the commandment "you shall have no other gods before me for I am the G-d who freed you from Egyptian bondage." An "idol of the cave" is perhaps not just an inanimate object that is worshiped as a substitute for G-d, but also perhaps the delusional belief that the "systems" no matter how inventive and sophisticatedly crafted by *techne*, are mere human products. Human beings construct or deconstruct to make systems. However only G-d uniquely creates out of nothing- *yesh miayin*. Avraham when he broke the idols of Terah's store according to the Midrash, and as the teacher of the world of ethical monotheism, understood the evil of idolatry (in all its forms) best.

Thus we return where this introduction began—with Avraham as the revealer of ethical monotheism. According to the Midrash this inner intuitive vision that lead to the unveiling of the logics of thought to demonstrate a perfect unique self sufficient creator sprung from the inner advice of the kidneys that taught Avraham the truth of ethical monotheism. Thus the Kidneys came to be associated in Rabbinic thought with *aitzah* or advice. In rabbinic texts the kidneys were thus associated with morality and ethical activity and the seat of conscience as Kopple has shown in his article "the Biblical view of the Kidney" (Am. J Nephrology 1994: 14: 279-281.

Kidneys in Rabbinic texts[45]

In general Rabbinic Judaism rejected the notion of the four humors so essential to Greek medicine. The four humors of the body for Greek medicine were: blood, yellow bile, phlegm, and black bile. Health involved the proper balance of the four humors while disease was a function of an imbalance of them. The rabbis considered that disease could be the result of structural disorders of internal organs. Most Talmudic sages attributed diseases either to environmental factors such as cleanliness or internal inherent causes. They saw a cause and effect relationship between improper diet, excess food, excessive heat or cold, uncleanliness, fear, worry, mental

---

[45] See Dvorjetski, E. The history of nephrology in the Talmudic corpus, Am J Nephrology 22, 119-129, 2002

anxiety, and infection as resulting in disease and even had notions of heredity responsible for carrying on certain traits for example when Jacob bred Lavan's sheep.[46] In a sugya (section) of the Talmud the rabbis also indicate hereditary factors with regards to a child who bled profusely at a *bris milah* (hemophilia) and how this appeared a generation later in the same related family subsequent generations.

The rabbis recognized that parasites can cause liver, lung, and intestinal damages and eating raw or inadequately cooked beef can cause tapeworm of the intestines. The rabbis argued that retention of bile causes jaundice as noted by JH Bass in *Outlines of the History of medicine* (Henderson HE, trans. York, 1889). The Rabbis of the Talmud knew that disease can be spread by contact with a diseased person, their food, water, secretions, or garments. The rabbis considered the color, consistency, position, growths on, and lessions of internal organs of sacrificed animals of goats, sheep, and cows. They described cavities and lessions on the lungs as suggesting lung disease (tuberculosis) which rendered an animal unfit to be eaten or trefa. Today in kashrut the shochet must examine the pleural cavity and the lung of a cow before declaring it suitable for food by moving the hand through the pleural cavity and inflating the lung by lowing through the trachea. The lungs must inflate completely so there is an absence of consolidation, fibrosis or cavities. Thus the rabbis made the connection between disease and changes in the structure of internal organs. In the 19th century Virchow and Cohnheim *apres la lettre* asserted the pathological basis of diseases as they pioneered pathological anatomy. These scientists credit the Talmudists as the

---

[46] Bogacz, Yoram, Experience, heredity and Yaakov Avinu's sheep, Dialogue 1,2 (2012) 32-50;

source of their insights according to SR Kagan in _Jewish Medicine_ (Boston: Independent Press, 1952).

Knowledge of the kidney as in talmudic times resulted from determining the suitability of animals for food which is the subject of a study by Drs Libovich and A Steinberg. The Talmudic sages understood that the excretion or lack thereof of urine could suggest disease. Thus reduction of urine output causes dropsy, suggesting that urine is a vehicle through which the water ingested by a person leaves the body. The rabbis for example noted that the urine of camels and horses is not thick and does not resemble milk. Therefore it is merely water coming into the body and exiting the body (cited by J. Preuss, *Biblical and Talmudic Medicine*, 1993). However the milk of an ass is milky and thick. Therefore it may contain parts of the body or exudations of the body. This intuits that the urine may remove from the body components besides water. Thus the rabbis saw urine serving the purpose of releasing excess water. And secondly expelling potential harmful toxins.

The Talmud refers to the "gate of the kidney" (*hilus*) employing the Hebrew word Haritz. In Maseket Hullin, chapt. 55, verse the small kidney makes the animal unsuitable for food or trefa. Subsequent post-Talmudic discussion considered if a small kidney makes animals trefa. Rashi (1040-1105) writes succinctly that disease is the cause of the small kidney phenomenon reasoning that disease shrinks and contracts the kidney. On the other hand Rabbi Nissim (14th C.) asserts that an animal can be born with a small kidney which is verified today as *aplasia*.These 2 factors are codified in Shulchan Aruch, Yoreh Deah (ch.44:5). It notes that a small kidney with scars on the surface and its covering cramped is the result of internal disease, but small kidney from birth that is smooth and its covering not cramped is congenital. Thus the animal with a small kidney, not the result of disease (has signs of scarring) is kosher. Richard Bright formalized and expanded on these rulings in the 19th century which had existed in Talmudic law long before, *apres la lettre*.

Shulchan Aruch (Yoreh Deah ch. 44: 4) observes a kidney with a *Shalphit* (cyst) filled with clear water.. This does not preclude the animal being suitable for food or kosher. Thus the rabbis are aware of the renal cyst as a benign condition. However a kidney with turbid water with an offensive smell makes an animal trefa (Shulchan Aruch, ch. 45, verse 6). This sounds like a renal abscess, a very serious condition. Also considered are bulls that urinate blood attributed to a rupture in the bladder... or a rupture in the kidney due to trauma. Thus rabbis knew that trauma can cause injury to the kidney or urinary tract what is called hematuria.

In summary, then Jewish medicine before the medieval ages is represented in the Bible which provides extensive principles for hygiene and prevention of diseases and codes for dietary regimes. Also anatomical examination is widely testified in tractates of the Talmud like Hullin with regards to the dissection of animals for the sake of determining their fitness or unfitness for eating as kosher. This examination of animal entrals lead to a pathological basis for understanding disease and the disease process. Thirdly observations by early rabbis on the presentation of various diseases is also documented in Rabbinic texts such as the Talmudim.

Medieval Jewish Physicians and the Kidneys

Any history of the Jews in Medicine is bound to mention five exemplary Jewish physicians. They are: Asaph Judaeus the son of Berekhayahu, Isaac Israeli or Isaac Judaeus, Maimonides, and the Paduan physician Bartholemaeus de Montagnano and the graduate of the

University of Padua Tovia Cohen. Whole books are written on these Jewish physicians so we cannot do justice to their contribution to medicine or nephrology for that matter. Let us briefly note some of the known facts surrounding them.

(a) *Sefer Harfuoth* is attributed to Asaph. Scholars such as Steinschneider[47], Loew, Friedenwald, Venetianer, Muntner, and Melzer have made arguments for his dates or in which century he lived with a range between the 3rd century in Persia to the 10th century. What we do know is that five manuscripts exist of *Sefer Harfuoth* namely: Munich 231, Oxford 2138, Florence, Paris, and British Museum (Gaster collection). The Munich codex is most complete at 553 pages. The work contains information on herbal remedies with their names provided in Hebrew, Greek, Latin, and Syriac. Reference to the use of magic in therapy is frowned upon. Also space is given to: (a) anatomical aspects of some internal organs, (b) nutrient values for foods such as milk and milk products, (c) various diseases prevalent during certain months of the year, (d) herbs for healing, (e) antidotes against disease, (f) the utility of uroscopy for diagnosis of diseases, (g) Hippocratic maxims. Asaph before William Harvey realized that blood circulates through vessels (*geedeem* in Hebrew) that originate in the heart, reach the far end of the body and from

---

[47] See Steinshneider, Moritz, Die hebraischen Ubersetzungen des Mittelalters und die Juden als Dolmetscher (Graz: Akademische Druck- u. Verlagsanstalt, 1956 (1893).

their return to the heart. He also knew that the origin of the egg and sperm uniting was the uterus long before the modern discipline of obstetrics.

With regard to nephrology Asaph used uroscropy and the value of the appearance of the urine in evaluating diseases and their prognosis. According to the Bible Asaph considered the kidney as the seat of thought and apprehension and humility.

(b) Isaac Israeli is Abu Yacob Ishak ibn Suleiman al Israeli. It is Isaac ben Solomon in Hebrew. His dates are roughly 832-932 or 850-950 CE. While in Egypt he was a famous ocultist he went to Kairwan as the court physician to Prince Ziyadat Allah and later the Caliph Obaid Allah). He wrote the following medical works:
   a. Kitab al Hummayat (Book of Fever)
   b. Ktab al Baul (Book on Urine analysis)[48]
   c. Kitab al Adwiyate al Mifradah wal Aghadia (Book on Remedies)
   d. Musar Harofim (Guidelines or ethics for physicians)

His books were subsequently translated into Hebrew, Latin, Spanish, and Italian. The Latin version was done

---

[48] See Collins, Kenneth, Historical Note: On the Glasgow Hebrew manuscript of Isaac's Book of Urine, Korot, vol 20, 2009-2010; The existence of the Hebrew ms of Isaac Israeli's Book of Urine, Sefer ha-sheten originally composed in Arabic as Kitav al-bawl in the Hunterian Collection of Glascow University Library is by Isaac Israeli (850-950) who wrote this work in Kairouan in modern Tunisia, where he studied around 907 CE and it remained a medical classic in European medical schools, after translation into latin by Constantinus Africanus.

from 1070 to 1078 by a monk from Monte Cassino named Constantine of Carthage.

Translation of texts from Hebrew into Latin and Arabic is also attested later in history by the Rector of the University of Leipzig who writes around 1518: "In the libraries of Jews, a treasure of medical science lies hidden, a treasure as scarce as is to found in other language. Nobody will be able to get access to this treasure without intimate knowledge of the Hebrew Grammar." (see Berger, N, "Why medicine? In Berger N (ed) *Jews and Medicine: Religion, Culture, Science*, Beth Hatefusoth, 1995, p.13-32). In the Renaissance Jews also translated Arabic and Hebrew writings into Latin which facilitated the migration of medical knowledge into Europe.

In Isaac Israel's book on Urine Analysis he includes the following sections:
- a. The science of urine
- b. Importance of night urine
- c. Different kinds of urine and their diseases
- d. Urine as the drainage of humor
- e. Different kinds of urine according to their color
- f. Colors showing the organ degradation
- g. Limpid / clear or muddy / thick honey like urines and their significance
- h. Urinary sediment in relation to pathology
- i. Kinds of urine in conjunction with sediment
- j. Other kinds of urine and sediments and their interpretations

(c) Maimonides 1135-1204. Rambam known as Rabbi Moshe ben Maimon wrote in the areas of halakah (*Sefer mishneh Torah and Pirush al -hamishnah*), philosophy (*sefer Moreh HaNekhim*), logic (*Sefer Hahigayon*), Music (Responsa on Listening to Music), Numerous letters to various communities (ie. *Letter to the Jews of Marseilles against engaging in Astrology*) and compositions such as the *Tractate on Ressureciton, Tracate on Apostasy,* etc as well as a large body of medical writings some of which has been edited by Dr. Fred Rosner. S.G. Massry wrote an article in the American Journal of Nephrology (1994: 14, 307-312) titled "Maimonides: Physician and nephrologist." Although too extensive to note in detail or any depth here, in regards to nephrology, Rambam's medical writings reference knowledge to body homeostatis, kidney function, obstruction of urinary tract, polyuria of diabetes mellitus, and diabetes insipidus, nephrotic syndrome, hemoglobinuria and or black water fever, proteinuria and indication of chronicity of illness, macroscopic hematuria as a reflection of glomerular disease and the use of sweating as a thereapeutic modality in conditions associated with urine retention.

Fred Rosner and Sussman Muntner have written on Maimonides's aphorisms regarding analysis of Urine. The collection of Rambam's aphorisms are presented in 25 chapters or treatises based on mainly the works of Galen. Each treatise deals with a different subspecialty in medicine. The fifth treatise contains aphorisms with lessons pertaining to the urine and its examination.[49]

The treatise on Urine opens:
> (1) It is obligatory to perform tests and to examine the urine during any fever because fevers are sicknesses occurring in vessels.

---

[49] I cite the following from Rosner, p. 43-98, 1983.

Therefore in pleuritis, one should first examine the sputum and afterwards to a urinalysis because pleuritis is not ordinarily one of the fever producing illnesses..... De Crisibus VI (I).

(2) The most propitious sediments of those which settle in the urine during fever following sepsis are those which arise from the liquid which already became putrefied by arteries which contained it. From this, evenly distributed white sediments develop which settle in the urine without spreading detestable odors (De Febribus I.)

(3) If the particles of the urinary sediment are all equal in appearance and in quality this signifies the dominance of nature over the illness and its rule over it (the patient will be cured). Urine in which foam (literarly air) accumulates is caused by cold liquids and therefore shows the chronicity of the illness (Comment. Aphroismorum VII).

(4) The most favorable urine in ill people is one which most closely resembles the urine of healthy individuals. Maximally cooked urine in the healthiest of people is urine which is even in thickness and whose yellowness leans to a tinge of redness to deepen the yellow color. This is because some moisture of blood and red bile become mixed into it (De Crisibus I).

(5) The most propitious type of urine is one with a nice appearance. It has a white turbidity in it which is flat and even and should it settle to bottom of a vessel, this is the best sign. IF it settles in the middle it is less favorable than the first. If it floats on top, it is less favorable than the second. These three types of urine are a measure of the

degree of cooking. Of the other types of urine, some demonstrate the opposite of cooking and some herald a catastrophy (De Crisibus I)- (Rosner notes that Aphorisms 3, 4, and 5 are laking in the Arabic manuscript but present in Hebrew and Latin).

(6) The evenness of sediments and their settling down set forth two conditions. One is that sediments not be dispersed and mixed with other particulate matter but remain compact, and secondly that they should remain so at all times because sometimes the urine is found to be clear at one time and at another time, settlings and sediment are seen in it. In such a case, the sediment found during urinalysis is not favorable since it is a sign that cooking was not completed. De Crisibus I

(7) The most favorable urines of patients (prognostically) are those which when micturated demonstrate the most favorable sediments fully cooked as just described because this signifies that nature has already triumphed over the illness and has begun to excrete the illness-producing liquids. After this in propitiousness is a urine which is micturated turbid but which settles out favorable sediments after standing awhile since this signifies that nature has commenced the activity of cooking and will soon complete this activity . After this second type of propitiousness is a urine which is micturated thick but then clears and no sediment forms at all. This signifies that the cooking time is far off even though nature has initiated efforts in this direction De Crisibus I.

(8) A sedmiment always occurs in the urine of those ill with fever which occurred during complete rest and relaxation and who increase their food intake at the end of the illness. However in those who get their fever following work and exercise the illness will often terminate without the occurrence of any sediment in the urine. They complete the cooking rapidly with the appearance of a white, flat and evenly distributed turbidity in the upper part of the urine or suspended in the middle De Crisibus I

(9) If illnesses occur secondary to favorable liquids, then urinary sediments will be plentiful. If these (illnesses) however originate from red liquids then no sediments at all will form or only very few. Comment. Prognostikon II

(10) The most unfavorable urine of all sick people is the thin, clear, one which resembles well water, uncolored and translucent. It is farthest from being cooked. Somewhat less dangerous is the urine which when micturated was thin and clear but after a short time becomes cloudy since this signifies that nature although behind in its task, will soon perform it. Less unfavorable than the second is urine which is micturated cloudy and remains cloudy because this shows that nature is as yet undecided and although it is attempting to cook, as yet has not accomplished anything De Crisbius I....[50]

---

[50] Maimonides, Moses, Studies in Judaica: The Medical Aphorisms of Moses Maimonides, Vol I, trans. And edited by Fred Rosner and Muntner Suessman, Bloch Publishing Co., p.- 93-98, 1973.

There are a total of 20 long paragraph notes by the Rambam relating to urinalysis in the fifth treatise. Readers should see this text translated into English by Rosner and Muntner published by Bloch Publishing Co. for Yeshivah University press, NY.

(d) University of Padua Jewish Medical Graduates

From the 11th to the 17th century Jews were not admitted to Christian European Universities in large numbers. Admission was highly restricted and often those who were allowed to attend did not often receive a degree at the end of their studentship.

An exception to this quota was the University of Padua that allowed Jewish students to study and awarded them degrees. 229 physicians graduated from the University between 1409 and 1721. Under the rule of the Carrara family, the University of Padua flourished in the 14th century. The first medical doctorate awarded a Jew was in 1409. Between 1517-1619 80 Jews graduated from the medical school in Padua. Between 1619 and 1721 149 Jews received degrees and the number increased to 325 by 1816. The University was sensitive to Jewish students. They did not have to have on their diploma the date referring to Christ and Jewish diplomas state *"In Dei Aeterni Nomine Amen"* in the name of the eternal God versus Christian diplomas that stated *In Christi Nomine Amen*. The date of the diploma was also adjusted for Jewish graduates. For example for a Jew the date might state *Currente Anno* while in a Christian diploma the dates stated *Anno a partu Virginis or Anno a Christi Nativitate*. However tuition was double for Jews and graduates were required to send tribute taxes to upkeep snacks for current students so they could eat meat and sweets.

During the Renaissance at the University of Padua the Church no longer was able to curtail autopsy and dissection of human corpses. The Church as with Rabbinic culture was concerned that autopsy would violate the sanctity of respecting the body divinely given to each born invidividual in God's plan.[51] Dissection provided detailed information on the structure of the various organs which was championed by scientists like Andreas Vesalius (1514-1564) and Realdo Colombo (1516-1559). (see De Broe ME, Sacre D. Snelder Ed, De Weert DI, Flemish anatomist Andreas Vesalius and the kidney, Am J. Neprhology 1997, 17:252-360 & Eknoyan, G de Santo NG "Realdo Colombo" a reappraisal, Am J Nephrology 1997: 17: 261-268). Besides dissection the microscope was invented at the end of the 16th century and permitted new discoveries. Further William Harvey (1578-1657) made break throughs in understanding the Circulatory system and Malphigh (1628-1694) described the renal corpuscle.

Among these University of Padua graduates were many Jews including: Joseph del Medigo, Salmon Congeliano, Tovia Cohen, Montagnano. *Modena and Morpurgo have published a list of Jewish medical graduates from Padua.*[52] Many Jews returned to their home towns after the curriculum in Padua. For instance De Jonases returned to practice medicine in Lemberg (Lvov), the Montaltos in Lublin, the de Limas and Wincklers in Posen, the Gordons in Vilna and Marpugos in Cracow, Del Medigo

---

[51] Misher, Jason, Autopsies in Jewish law : a dissection of the sources., ורפא ירפא 3 (2011) 111-129 ; Washofsky, Mark, On the absence of method in Jewish bioethics : Rabbi Yehezkel Landau on autopsy, Jewish Law Association Studies 17 (2007) 254-278; Jakobovits, Immanuel,Sir, Halakhic debate on brain death., Le'ela 41 (1996) 29-30.

[52] *"Medici Churghli Ebrei Dottorate e Licenziate nell Universita di Padova dal 1617 al 1816*, Bologna, Forni Editori, 1617 pp

practiced in Vilna, Frankfurt, and Prague (see Friedenwald, H, The Jews in Medicine KTAV, 1994, 253-256)

(i)   Tovia Cohen (1652- 1729)[53] made contributions to the field of nephrology. In his book, *Ma'aseh Toviah* he examines uroscopy, kidney function, body fluid homeostasis, and obstructive uropathy. His book appeared in 1708 and the preface was written by Salmon Conegliano (1642-1719) a noted and important physician himself, also a graduate of the University of Padua. The book is an encyclopedic work in 138 pages, in two parts. Part II constitutes sections on medicine, hygiene, medical botany, and secret diseases such as syphilitic afflictions, and one section discourses on diseases of the "closed garden" (reference to *Song of Songs*) dealing with gynecological and obstetrical diseases. Another is titled "disease of the fruit of the body" that is in the area of pediatrics. The book likens the human body to a house. The hair is the roof. The ears the corners of the roof.

---

[53] Massry, Shaul, "Jewish Medicine and the University of Padua: Contributions to the Padua Graduate Toviah Cohen to Nephrology," *American Journal of Nephrology* 19:2 (1999) p. 213-221. I cite all factoids and extensively from Massry's article.

The eyes the windows. The mouth the door. The liver and spleen are the middle story where cooking occurs and the spleen is the cellar. The Kidney is the water well that provides vital water to the house and the lower intestines are the bathroom and toilets. The feet are the foundation of the house.

Tovia Cohen's Contribution to neprhology:

Tovia defines the urine as a juice derived from the blood and generated by the kidney from drinking liquids and eating moist foods. This shows Tovia knows that the urine is secreted or filtered by the kidney from the blood. Galen made similar remarks. Also Tovia understands that water and fluid intake is the source of urine. Tovia also knows that the urinary system is required for the maintenance of the body and this system may be hurt by diseases and thus he understand the urinary system as essential for a proper balance of homeostatis. Tovia also makes observations on the importance of a physician to examine the urine as did Maimonides. Like Maimonides he notes that the urine's constitution, appearance, volume, color, and odor provide important signs to the various ailments of someone with kidney disease. This led Tovia to provide 10 cautionary caveats to ensure the accuracy of urinalysis which are:

(1) The urine must be sampled once and not many times
(2) This must be in the morning on an empty stomach when food is digested
(3) The urine should be taken in a clear transparent pumpkin shaped vessel

(4) The container should be covered and kept in a warm place in order to protect it from cold and heat and direct sunlight

(5) The urine must not be observed less than 1 hour after sampling

(6) It must not be observed later than 6 hours which is the time limit for observing the cloudiness and components

(7) If during the time the urine is altered due to an external or internal cause, the container should be immersed in a cup of water so that the urine may resume its original form

(8) Observation of the urine must be performed in a well lighted place but not in direct sunlight

(9) Urine must not be sampled after drinking wine, nor after eating saffron, asparagus, or taking medication like rhubarb which alters urine

(10) In fearing that urine may be altered by exposure to air or to sunlight the physician should place his hand on the side of the container facing the sun to serve as a barrier between the sun and the container

Further Tovia was very perceptive about the impact of the amount or volume of urine output. A normal amount of urine volume indicates that the amount of urine is in proportion to the amount of fluid intake. Large urine output suggests wetness of the body (overhydration) and small volume denotes dryness of the body or excess aspiration (dehydration). This speaks to fluid homeostasis and the role of the kidney in this process.

Tovia also describes the physiology of the bladder. He notes it is made of two skins (tunica or layers) one with the force which draws and the other with the force which propels the urine into the two tubes from the kidneys to the bladder. He raised for the first time vesicoureteral reflux through the foce of the muscular layer of the bladder to propel urine back into the ureters.

Tovia described the following four ailments that may effect the urinary tract:

(a) Urinary retention which is due to blood clots, thick mucus, excess spirit, stone, verruca or polyp. This causes renal pain (colic) which is different from abdominal pain (pain in intestines). There may be a delay (oliguria) or shut down (anuria) of urine.

(b) Tovia recommends for kidney stones drinking tea made of certain herbs that are capable of promting diuresis and breaking down the stones

(c) The 2nd ailment of the urinary system is hesitancy of urination (dysuria in Latin and burning in german). There are 3 signs
   a. Urine drips like boiling water
   b. Pain is experienced during urination before and after
   c. It is due to fever of the kidneys and bladder (urinary tract infection) and at time stone in bladder.

Tovia proposes the use of drugs that cool and cleanse the bladder to treat infection and the patient should drink barley water, herbal tea, and juices.

(d) Dripping of the urine (cold disease in German) is a condition caused by coldness of the abdomen and at times of sour mucus. It is called dripping since the patient gives one drop and stops then a second and third drop all with pauses between drops. This ailment may be due to enlargement of the prostate or urethra.

(e) Polyuria denotes continuous urination with no ability to stop and is called in Latin Diabetes which has 2 characteristics
   a. Clear without any change (dilute urine)
   b. White and clear

As Massry concludes in summary Toviah's nephrology knowledge was quite advanced for the time although Jeremy Brown notes Cohen rejected Copernicus' findings in astronomy.[54] He knew about the importance of fluid intake, urinary output, body fluid homeostasis and the effect of overhydration and dehydration on urine volume, the role of the kidney in this fluid homeostatis, treatment of kidney stones, and four ailments that effect the urinary system including UTI,

---

54 See Library guide by David B Levy at http://libguides.tourolib.org/scienceandtorah article, "The Structure of Scientific Revolutions" (Kuhn) in Astronomy " by DBL based on work of Jeremy Brown and Thomas Kuhn. See Brown, Jeremy, New Heavens, and a New Earth: : The Jewish Reception of Copernican Thought, Oxford University Press, 2012 ; Tuvia Cohen in Ma'aseh Tuviah called Copernicus "the son of Satan". Cohen's review of astronomy is found in his work, Olam Hagalgulim (the world of spheres). While Cohen had accepted the revolution in biology by acknowledging the truth of William Harvey's work on the Circulation of the blood he rejected Copernicus. Tuvia placed more importance on medicine than astronomy. Yet astronomical knowledge was seen as a good to help explaining the laws of the lunar cycle and luach (hilkhot kiddush hahodesh) while related mathematical knowledge such as Euclid's geometry and later Algebra was helpful for clarifying tractates like Maseket Eruvin. T.B. Shabbat 75a commenting on the pusek: "For this is your wisdom and understanding among the nations" (Deut. 4:6) concluded that it referred to the "calculation of the seasons and the constellations" that is the ability to create an accurate calendar, and to forecast the position of the stars and planets, etc.

obstruction , urinary hesitancy (infection), and polyuria. He provided an insightful clinical differential diagnosis between renal and abdominal colic. He raised the possibility that the bladder may participate in the genesis of vesicoureteral reflux. For more on Jewish thought and scientific discovery in the Early modern Europe see David Ruderman (Yale University Press, 1995).

Toviah practiced in Cracow, Adrinopole, Constantinople, and is buried in Jerusalem. Tovia's grandfather was from Safed and came to Crakow and was a rabbi and physician. Tovia's father was Moshe Cohen and practiced medicine in Noral Poland and then fled the persecutions of the Cossacks during Tach VeTat in 1648 to practice in Metz France. Initially Tovia got permission with his friend Gabriel Felix to attend the University of Frankfurt an der Oder with permission of Frederick Wilhelm I, Grand Elector of Brandenburg. Then Tovia enrolled in the University of Padua in 1681 and graduated 2 years later in 1683. After medical school he went back to Cracow and then to Adrianope and then Constantinople where with the support of Prince Maurocordata and the great Vazir Rumi Pasha he served as the court physician to Sultan Ahmad II.

(d) Paduan physician such as Bartholomaeus de Montagnano

    (ii)   A famous painting attributed to Gerrit Dou (17th C) represents a Jewish physician perhaps Montalto (d 1616, buried in Amsterdam), a Jewish physician to the court of Marie de Medicis and Louis XIII, examining a flask of urine while utilizing the book of Isaac Israeli on urine analysis. Thus the flask or vessel called in the middle ages, the *matula*, for examining urine became a symbol of the medical profession. In antiquity uriscopy was associated with divination to diagnosis. Urinalysis is essential to the fields of urology, endocrinology, nephrology which uses clearance studies to make important conclusions about the health of persons suffering form kidney diseases. The painting of Montagnano is the contextual legacy of todays tools of medicine in the proteomic profiling and detection of biomarkers in the urine.

History of Nephrology in Non-Jewish World: Antiquity to Medieval to Renaissance[55]

ANCIENT

Ancient Mesopotamia[56]

---

[55] Greydanus DE, Sankar Raj VM, Merrick J (2015) A Short Historic View of Nephrology upto the 20th Century . Clinics Mother ChildHealth 12: 195. doi: 10.4172/2090-7214.1000195 Page 3 of 7Clinics Mother Child HealthISSN:2090-7214 CMCH, an open access journal Volume 12 • Issue 4 • 1000195

[56] Hogg, HW, "Heart and Reins in ancient Literature of the Near East, J Manchester Univ Egyptian Oriental Soc 1, 49-91, 1911

Basic knowledge of medical conditions is traced to Mesopotamia (3100 BCE to 332 BCE) that included Sumer[57] and the Akkadian, Babylonian,[58] and Assyrian empires in modern-day Iraq and in antiquity in general.[59] Scholars who have looked at cuneiform clay tablets[60] of this enchorial era and identify references to descriptions reflective of urinary obstruction, urethritis (and urethral discharge), renal stones, and cysts. Archaic models of a kidney have been found such as that from the 13th century BCE found at an ancient temple in Kition, Cyprus; this bronze artifact has been interpreted by scholars as an example of an offering (*"ex voto suscepto* or from the vow made"*) to the temple gods by a person with kidney disease or as a teaching aid by the euhemerists or priest doctors of the temple. Babylonian physicians based diagnoses on the appearance of urine (i.e., beet juice, wine, beer, paint, others) and therapy of renal or genitourinary conditions was with local remedies from indigenous plants or minerals and

---

[57] Kramer, Samuel Noah, History Begins at Sumer, Garden City, N.Y. : Doubleday, 1959

[58] Jastrow, M: The medicine of Babylonians and Assyrians, Proc Roy Soc Med 7: 109-176, 1914; Geller MJ, & Cohen SL, Kidney and urinary tract disease in Ancient Babylonia, with trans. Of the cuneiform sources Kidney Interntional 47, 1811-1815, 1995

[59] See: Dhorme P, The metaphorical use of the names of body parts in Hebrew and Akkadiar, Revue Biblique 32, 489-517, 1922; Maio, G, The metaphorical and mythical use of the kidney in antiquity. Am J Nephrology 19: 101-106, 1999; Frazer JG, "Hearts and reins" and ideas of uncultured races, J. Manchester Univ. Egyptian Oriental Soc 1: 107-108, 1911; Geller, MJ: Die Babylonysch-assyriche Mediizin in Texten und Untersuchungen 7, In Rneal and Rectal Disease- Texts, Berlin Walter de Gruytren GMBH & Co 2005

[60] Chiera, Edward, They wrote on Clay, Chicago, Ill., The University of Chicago press,1938

blowing chemicals into the urethra; also, alcohol served as an anesthetic.

<u>Insights of Egyptology[61]</u>

"Homage to thee, O my heart! Homage to you, O my kidneys.!"

(Book of the Dead-8)[62]

Egyptian mummies reveal evidence of renal disease including renal stones and cysts. The Ebers Papyrus (1550 BCE) from ancient Egypt; it recommends a remedy for fluid retention (dropsy) that involves smearing on these patients a concoction made from cooked old papyri documents in oil. Unfortunately, there is only exiguous documentation on renal disease available to modern scholars from this time though there is some identified information about urinary retention, frequency, dysuria, and particularly red urine. Hematuria was etiologically linked, then, as now, in Egypt particularly from infection implanted in the bladder wall. The Egyptian *"Book of the Dead* (1600 BCE-1240 BCE) was revered by ancient Egyptians to help those in the after life[63] and was an early work to link the kidney with the heart. The heart

---

[61] Am J Nephrol. 1999;19(2):140-7.The kidney in ancient Egyptian medicine: where does it stand? Salem ME[1], Eknoyan G

[62] Budge, EAW, The Egyptian Book of the Dead. The Papyrus of Ani, NY: Dover Pub Inc. 1967

[63] Leca, A: The Egyptian Way of Death. Mummies and the Cult of the Immortal, Garden City, NY, Doubleday and Co Inc, 1981

and kidneys[64] were the only organs extracted in the process of mummification.[65]

KIDNEYS IN ANCIENT GREEK CIVILIZATION[66]

Aristotle in Histor. Animals Book 3 chapter 17:88[67] and Plinius in Histor. Natur. 11:81 put forward that animals have the most fat in the area of the kidneys. For this reason perhaps Isaiah (34:6) notes, "the sword of the L-rd is filled with blood. Of the fat of the kidneys of rams":

חֶרֶב לד' מָלְאָה דָם, הֻדַּשְׁנָה מֵחֵלֶב, מִדַּם כָּרִים וְעַתּוּדִים, מֵחֵלֶב כִּלְיוֹת אֵילִים: כִּי זֶבַח לד' בְּבָצְרָה, וְטֶבַח גָּדוֹל בְּאֶרֶץ אֱדוֹם

The medical school of Knidos (in Asia Minor) and its chief member Euryphon were interested in the systematic classification of diseases according to the systems involved. Galen[68] mentions that Knidian physicians were familiar with four renal diseases, probably the same described in the book *About Inner Sufferings,* whose author is not known with certainty;

---

[64] Salem, ME Eknoyan G: The kidney in ancient Egyptian medicine, Where does it stand? Am J. Nephrology 19:140-147, 1999

[65] Smith, GE, Heart and Reins in mummification, J Manchester Univ Egpytian Oriental Soc 1:41-44, 1911

[66] See Am Journal of Nephrology 1994;14(4-6):264-9. Hippocratic medicine and nephrology. Marketos SG.

[67] Aristotle considered the kidneys to be mere accessories of the bladder, which he thought was the main organ for the secretion of urine. Arisottle does however state (Hist. Anim. 1:7) that "the kidneys are suited to serve in the excretion of the fluit which collects in the bladder."

[68] Eknoyan, G, Origins of Nephrology, Galen, the founding father of experimental renal physiology, Am J. Nephr 966-82, 1989

Most investigators attribute it to the Knidian school (5th century BC), while others consider it to be a Hippocratic work. The first renal disease described in the book is nephrolithiasis with renal colic. The second disease corresponds to renal tuberculosis, while the remaining two are somewhat unclear; the third resembles either renal vein thrombosis or bilateral papillary necrosis. The fourth disease, described in the greatest detail of all, corresponds to a chronic suppurative renal infection or a sexually transmitted urethritis, complicated by renal involvement. Treatments described include: diet modification, physical exercise, ingestion of herbal extracts and surgery, as a last resort.

Later, Galen established the relationship between the kidneys and the making of urine. As Eknoyan shows, Galen relocated the site of making of urine from the bladder to the kidneys.[69] Galen refers to deposits or sediment in the urine as *paruphistamenon*. Cloudy urine is refered to as *nephele*. The Greek text explains *the paruphistamenon* as that thing in the urine which has different appearances (*heteron ti emphainon*) that manifest or appear (*emphainon*). Urine has consistency (*sustasis*) and color (*chroia*). Consistency is classified as having either thin, thick, or medium types. Some ascribe this shift in understanding also to Aretaeus.[70] While Hippocratic medicine based on rational thought and clinical observation investigated the speciality of nephrology, five centuries later Aretaeus of Cappadocia explored further in his writings the anatomy and

[69] Eknoyan, G the origins of nephrology: Galen the founding father of experimental renal physiology" in the *Am Journal of Nephrology* (1989: 9, 66-82

[70] Aretaeus, De Morbis Chronicis II, 3 ("On the diseases of the Kidneys") The original work was written in Greek. See the Extant works of Aretaeus (Fr. Adams, ed. & trnas.) London, 1856, p. 340-343

physiology from the Alexandrian school of Medicine. He wrote two books on acute and and two books on chronic diseases. He also addressed treatment of kidney disease. He considered herb therapy as a method for treating kidney disease. Book 2 chapter 3 of Aretaeus extensively describes kidney disease, particularly the affections of the kidneys [*De causis et signis acutorum morborum (lib. 2)* (ed. Francis Adams LL.D.)] including kidney stones.

Hippocrates was associated with the medical school of Kos. This school of medicine put emphasis on description of symptoms, prognostic implications, and treatment. Hippocrates also describes the formation of kidney stones in part 9 of *De aere aquis et locis* In Aphorism chapter 5 part 59 Hippocates writes, "Strangury supervenes upon inflammation of the rectum, and of the womb, and strangury supervenes upon *suppuration of the kidney*, and hiccup upon inflammation of the liver." In Prognostics ch 12 of Hippocrates we read,

> "So long as the urine is thin and of a yellowish red color, it is a sign that the disease is unconcoted and if the disease should also be protracted, while the urine is of this nature, there is a dangers lest the patient will not be able to hold on until the disease is concocted (trans Jones 2:27).[71]

---

[71] This passage from Hippocrates influenced the book of Remedies of Asaf [chaptes 471-72] when we see the paralle text of the later Asafian wording: And if you see that the urine is very much red, and it is thin- there is no oily dirt in it- until that disease becomes harsh, and then he cannot subdue it, because it (The disease) stands in its strength, And if the urine continues to be red and thin, know that his disease has defetated him and it will dominate the body until it has no strength to stop the power of the disease. (Munter "Asaf ha-rofe", Korot 4:550

Anatomy of the kidneys showed the relationship of the kidneys to the ureters. The first medical text on diseases of the kidneys and bladder was by Rufus of Ephesus (ca 1st CE) published a century before Galen.[72] Galen later described the anatomy of the kidney which he says he learned from examining the work of a butcher. Galen writes in book 1 part 13, "but practically every butcher is aware of this, from the fact that he daily observes both the position of the kidneys and the duct (termed the ureter) which runs from each kidney into the bladder, and from this arrangement he infers their characteristic use and faculty. But, even leaving the butchers aside, all people who suffer either from frequent dysuria or from retention of urine call themselves "nephritics," when they feel pain in the loins and pass sandy matter in their water."

In ancient Greece, Ephesus was not only a center for medical healing but also theater as Aristotle in *the Poetics*,[73] notes that watching a tragedy that has a turning point (perapetia) where the hero goes from happiness (eudaemonia) to unhappiness (a-eudamonia) would bring about a catharsis likened to a medical purification in the spectator. Thus the Greeks saw medicine and theater as intricately related and thus founded perhaps the first notion of the medical Humanities, although the Humanities as a discipline or field arose from the 16th Century Renaissance in Italy.

---

[72] Eknoyan, G, "Rufus of Ephesus and his diseases of the kidneys," Nephron 91, 383-392, 2002

[73] While the poetics looks at the anatomy of the tragedies of Aeschylus, Sophicles, and Euripides apparently Aristotle wrote an analysis of Greek Comedy as well that for some time was deposited in the Alexandrian Library, however the analysis of Comedy has been lost.

A fascinating study of Galen and Hippocrates the founding patriarchs of ancient Greek medicine and the Jews recently has appeared by Geller that is well worth the effort.[74]

While Galen (131-200 CE) did anatomical autopsy on monkeys it was Herophilus (300 BCE) of the Alexandrian school of medicine[75] (established in 332 BCE) which dissected dead bodies and Erasistratus also claims to have examined anatomical dissections of human bodies. In the Babylonian Talmud it was said that a disciple of Rabbi Ishmael dissected the body of a criminal women executed by the Romans, in the first century CE.

In ancient Greece and Rome infections of the kidney were described (*pyelonephritis*, absecess of the kidney, etc) which caused described symptoms such as pyuria, pain and fever. However most diseases of the renal parenchyma were unknown. It was thought up to the Renaissance that edema related to disease of the liver. Not to rehash already done work of a substantive time-line for the history of nephrology from antiquity on, the reader can find one at: http://www.era-edta.org/history/A_Timeline_of_the_History_of_Nephrology.pdf

This is a joint project of The International Association for the History of Nephrology.

---

[74] Geller, MJ, Hippocrates, Galen, and the Jews: Renal medicine in the Talmud, Am. J Nephrology 22, 101-106, 2002. Also of great interest is Shul Massry's article, "Influence of Judaism and Jewish Physicians on Greek and Byzantine Medicine and their Contribution to Nephrology," which appeared in *The American Journal of Nephrology* 17:3-4 (1997) p. 233-240.

[75] Kottek, SS Alexandrian medicine in the Talmudic Corpus, Korot 12: 80-89 1996-97

The ERA/EDTA And the Panhellenic Society for the History and Archaeology of Medicine By Athansios Diamandopoulos. This work treats the developments in knowledge of the kidney and its workings from Greek antiquity to the 14th century CE. The author index spotlights the views of the following thinkers:

AUTHOR INDEX [76]
1. Hippocrates, 5th cent. BCE
2. Aristotle, 4th cent. BCE
3. Erasistratus, 3rd cent. BCE
4. Philo Judeus 1st cent. BCE-1st cent. CE
5. Dioscurides, 1st cent. CE
6. Galen, 1st - 2nd cent. BCE
7. Rufus Ephesus, 1st - 2nd cent. CE
8. Arêtes Cappadociensis, 2nd cent. CE
9. Pseudo-Galen, 2nd cent. CE
10. Alexander Aphrodisiensis, 2nd-3rd cent. CE
11. Oribasius Pergamenus, 4th cent. CE
12. Nemesius of Emesa, 4thcent. CE
13. Palladius, 5th cent. CE
14. Alexander of Tralles, 6th cent. CE
15. Aetius Amidenous, 6th cent. CE
16. Stephanus of Alexandria, 7th cent. CE
17. Paul of Aegina, 7th cet. CE
18. Theophilus Protospatharius, 7th cent CE (?)
19. Stephanus of Athens, 9th-10th cent CE (?)
20. Damascius, 9th-10th cent CE (?)
21. Michael Psellus, 11th cent. CE
22. Symeon Seth, 11th cent. CE
23. Johannes Apocaucus, 13th cent. CE
24. Nicolaus Myrepsus, 13th cent. CE

---

[76] See J R Soc Med. 1993 May;86(5):290-3. **Acute renal failure according to ancient Greek and Byzantine medical writers.** Marketos SG[1], Eftychiadis AG, Diamandopoulos A.

25. Johannes Zacharias Actuarius, 13th cent. CE
26. Nicephorus Vlemmydes, 14th cent. CE

Medieval 13th Century Nephrological Texts

One of the major discoveries in 1952 of a medieval 13th century manuscript from the Chilandear monastery (Mount Athos, Greece) written in Old Serbian Slavonic language has uncovered the *Chilanar Medial Codex*. The oldest part is a text on uroscopy written in the 13th century or 14th century and consists of 35 text pages in 62 paragraphs. This text contains detailed descriptions of urine characteristics (color, consistency, sediment, odor, etc). It gives a Hippocratic description of urine formation from the filtration of metabolic and waste materials involving the four humors rather than blood and fumes (toxic metabolits) according to the theory of Theophilus, Protospatharius, and Isaac Israeli. The bladder is described as an organ for urine collection. There are about 100 descriptions of the kidney and urinary tract diseases and disorders. Symptoms and syndromes such as hematuria, dysuria, pyuria, renal colic, anuria, polyuria, edema and dropsy, urine retention, and fever are described in the context of clinical pictures of lithiasis of the kidney and or bladder, pyelonephritis, cystitis, necrotic renal disease indicative of renal tuberculosis and tumors, acute and chronic nephritus, renal failure and gout. Pharmacological prescriptions are simple herbal medicines given as renal ailments.[77]

RENAISSANCE

During the Renaissance anatomical examination via autopsy became an area that the Church was unable to

---

[77] see GS Gorieva, "Kidney disease in medieval Serbian ms from the chilandar moastery (Mount Athos, Greece) in J Neprhol 2006 (may-June 19 Suppl 10: 830-7

prevent as they tried in the medieval ages. Galen had done anatomy studies on monkeys. The founder of pathological anatomy, Morgagni (Giovanni Battista Morgagni: 1682-1771) described various renal disorders via autopsy.

Paracelsus (Theophrastus Bombastus von Hohenheim: 1493-1541), a physician from Switzerland, wrote about proteinuria, hematuria, gout, and edema; his preeminent work was the forerunner of using specific gravity in urinalysis. Edema (oedema) was originally called dropsy, a word first recorded in the penultimate decade of the 13th century and later connected to renal disease in the 19th century (vida infra). The father of anatomy, Andreas Vesalius (1514-1564), born in Brussels, Belgium, illustrated renal anatomy in his seminal work, *De Humani Corporis Fabrica* (1543).

The father of microscopic anatomy, Marcello Malphighi (1628-1694), identified the glomerulus (Malpighian corpuscle) and in 1666 published his observations on the kidney (and other organs) in *De viscerum structura exercitatio anatomica*. He wrote about the pyramids of the renal medulla and collecting ducts as well as other microscopic aspects of the kidney; use of dye injection led him to describe glomeruli as "...hanging like apples from the blood vessels, which, swollen with the black fluid, look like a beautiful tree."

Other anatomic scholars continued to advance the knowledge of this organ called the reins, such as the Italian Lorenzo Bellini (1748-1795: Bellini's ducts) in his Exercitatio *Anatomica de StructuraUsu Renum* (1662), the Russian Alexander Schumlansky (1748-1795: *De Structura renum* in 1782), and the Englishman William Bowman (1816-1892); Physiological Anatomy and Physiology of Man-1857 with Robert Bentley Todd) , and many other sages of science and medicine.

A Short Historic View of Nephrology upto the 20th Century (PDF Download Available) online.[78]

A summary of the discoveries in Nephrology and the allied field of urology from antiquity to the modern period can be summarized in chart format at follows:

Time Line Chart Ancient to Medieval and Renaissance Schematic Summary

Cuneiform uroscopic texts (ca 3200 BCE-332 BCE) in Sumer and the Akkadian Babylonian and Assyrian empires inmodern day Iraq	Neo-Assrian clay tables; see Markham J Geller, Renal and Rectal Disease Texts, Die babblonisch-Assyrische Medizin in Texten und Untersuchungen 7 (Berlin: Walter de Gruyter, 2005, 7-71, 250-51; see also: Akkadian Diagnostic Handbook ca 1700 BCE in Markham J Geller, Ancient Babylonian Medicine: Theory and Practice (Oxford: Wiley-Blackwell, 2010), 42 and 90-91
Coan Prenotions	A book earlier than Hippocrates; ; see Potter, Paul ed. And trans., Loeb Classical Library 9 (Cambridge, Mass: Harvard Univ Press, 2010) 103-270

[78] https://www.researchgate.net/publication/288871307_A_Short_Historic_View_of_Nephrology_upto_th e_20th_Century [accessed Mar 16 2018].

Hippocrates of Kos (460-370 BCE)	(born c. 460 bce, island of Cos, Greece—died c. 375 BCE, Larissa, Thessaly) ; Uroscopy texts in Aphorisms 7:31-35; Prognosticus ch 12; and Airs, Waters, Places ch.9; attention to substance and sediments of urine (less attention to color); "Bubbles appearing on the surface of the urine indicates disease of the kidneys and a prolonged illness.... Colorless urine is bad... the sudden appearance of blood in the urine indicates that a small renal vessel has burst (Corpus Hippocraticum, in Dunea G History of Nephrology: beginnings Hektoen International J Med Humanities)
Areteus of Capadocia (81-138 CE)	Known for his descriptions of diabetes (melting away of flesh into urine) and commented on anemia from renal insufficiency, renal colic, hydronephrosis, and other renal pathalogy
Pedanius Dioscorides (40-90 CE)	Formulated De Materia Medica (On Medical Material) ca 60 CE that became the standard encyclopedic pharmacopoeia of herbs and medicines from mid 1st C to the Renaissance; In this 5 volume set wrote about herbs to treat renal disease such as mallow for renal failure

Andromachus the Elder from Crete (ca 50 CE)	Looking for the therics or catholicons to cure the ailments of mankind, suggested mixing various drug conconctions to treat renal disease
Galen (130-201 CE)	Κλαύδιος Γαληνός; September 129 CE – ca. 200/ca. 216 ; Commentaries on Hippocrates; views on urine in ch.12 of the first book in his *De crisibus; attention to substance (ousia) and sediments of Urine (less attention to color); concluded that the kidney's clear blood; as a surgeon he showed that urine flows from the kidneys to the bladder (contra Aristotle) by performing ligation of the ureters*
Oribasius (326-403 CE)	First used term ureter and galvanized renal physiology by suggesting that urine was absorbed from the blood circulation by the kidneys

Jewish physicians with non-Galenic perspectives

Late Antiquity, Hippocratic influence; The Neoplatonic philosopher Damascius of the first half of the 6th C later in history mentions a Jewish physican called Domnus who wrote commentaries on the Works of Hippocrates in Greek (see Menachem Stern, Greek and Latin Authors on Jews and Judaism (Jerusalem:The Israel Academy of Science and Humanities, 1974), 1:368-69; 2:679; Geller, MJ, Hippocrates, Galen and the Jews: Renal Medicine in the Talmud Am J. Nephr 22: 101-106, 2002

Anonymous early medieval uroscopic texts attributed apocraphally to Galen and Hippocrates

See: Gundolf KJeil, "Die Urognostische Praxis in vor-und fruehsalernitansicher Zeit (Habiltationischrift, Albert-Ludwigs-Universitat, Freiburg in Breisgau, 1970), 19-41; Baader, "Early Medieval Latin Adaptations," 255-56; Faith Wallis, "Signs and Senses: Diagnosis and Prognosis in Early Medieval Pulse and Urine Texts," Social History of Medicine 13 (2000): 265-78; Wallis, "Inventing Diagnosis: The ophilus De Urinis in the Classroom," DYNAMIS: Acta hispanica ad medicinae scientiarumque historiam illustrandam 20 (2000): 31-73.

Indian Medical Texts	4rth and 5th C CE; Caraka Samhita and the Susruta Samhita in Sanskrit

6th C CE, Book of Remedies (Sefer ha-refu'ot), Byzantine Empire; references Book of Jubilees; familiar with Rabbi Moshe Ha-Darshan of 11th C Provence; Content includes (a) Hippocrates Prognostics commentary (b) Hippocrates Aphorisms, (c) Dioscorides' Materia Medica.;Immanuel Low and Moritz Steinschneider argued for influence of Syraic texts particularly pharmaceutical topics influenced it- a 13th C report by Gregory Bar Hebraeus a Jewish physician called Masarjawayh, translated a syriac medical encyclopedia composed by Ahrun into Arabic around 684 CE ; See Suessman Muntner, ed. "Asaf ha-rofe Sefer Refu'ot (Asaf the Physician, Book of Remedies), Korot 3 (1965: 396-422, 533-60; 4 (1968: 11-40, 170-207, 389-443; 531-72, 691-730; 5 no 1 (1971): 27-68, 160-87, 295-330; 5 no 2 (1971-72): 435-73, 603-49, 773-807; 6, no 1 (1972):28-51 (based on Oxford ms); Ronit-Yoeli-Tlalim is working on a critical edition; Muntner, "asaf ha-rofe" Korot 3:408-9); Venetianer, Asaf Judaeus; For example in the Book of Remedies 498.7 (Muntner, Asaf ha-rofe, Korot 4:557) we read: יש השתן הלבן רבים אותותאיו

Asaf son Berakhyahu *In Tehillim Asaf ben Berakhyahu authored some Psalms; Rashi's commentary on Shoftim 15:15 contains one of the earliest references to the Book of Remedies. וַיִּמְצָא לְחִי-חֲמוֹר, טְרִיָּה; וַיִּשְׁלַח יָדוֹ וַיִּקָּחֶהָ, וַיַּךְ-בָּהּ אֶלֶף אִישׁ Rashi comments: טְרִיָּה: Moist. I saw in a **book of cures** that the moisture which issues from a wound is called טְרִיָּה

שתן לבן אשר יגיד על ריוון הכוח כי רוב שתן הזקנים לבן ושתן הגופים הקרים לבן ויש מן השתן הלבן אשר יגיד כי יש בגוף ההוא חולי מרוב ימים וגידי הגוף מסותמים ויש אשר יקרא בחולי ההוא מרוב משתה היין וכשר תראה השתן עב ולבן דע כי נמס אחד היסורים אשר הגביר על הגוף ותחל הרפואה

Asaf is noting that urine has many signs and kinds of diseases. There is white urine which tells the weakness of the power, because the urine of most elderly people is white, and the urine of cold bodies is white. And some of the white urines indicate that there is a disease in the body for a longer time and the veins of the body are blocked And some white urine occur in that sickness which is due to drinking of wine. And if you see that the urine is thick and white, know that one of the elements (yesodim) which

Yochanan (some chapters of Sefer ha-refu'ot attributed to Yochanan son of Zbdh (Zabda) from Jericho (yrhni); Likely Asaf and Yohanan belonged to the same intellectual circles which consisted of physicians who were interested in Hippocrates writings but preferred Hebrew as the language of learning

6th-7th C CE Disciple of Asaf, teich Book of Remedies, cited therein; Chapter 3 of the Book of Remedies divides the human body into 12 departments (mahlaqot), 248 members (avarim), and 365 veins. This parallels the Mishnah that enumerates 248 members of the body," האיברין אין להן שיעור אפי' פחות מכזית מן המת ופחות מכזית מן הנבילה ופחות מכעדשה מן השרץ מטמאין טומאתן " The Targum Yonathan mentions 365 nerves (giddin) along with 248 members. A well known gematria in the Bavli adds 248 (positive mitzvoth)+ 365 (negative mitzvoth, and also the days of the year) to arrive at 613 or the TaRYaG ha-mitzvot (see Makkot 23b)

Magnus of Emesa

6th C CE; distinguished six colors of urine and their prognostic values; Greek source of Magnus of Emesa's treatise was transmitted in 3 versions attributed to Galen: (a) De signis ex urinis edited by Paul Moraux, (b) De urinis (c) De urinis compendium printed in Kuehn's edition fo Galens Opera omnia and also by Ideler's Physici et medici Graeci minors; Another version translated into Latin as Liber medicine orinalibus attributed to Hermogenes. Survives in abbey of Montecassion see UC Bussemaker, "Ueber Magnus von Emesis und dessen Buch von Harne," Janus 2 (1847): 273-97; Bussemaker, "Traite d'Etienne su les urine publie pour le premiere foois d'apres un manuscript de la Biblioheque roale," Revue de philogie, de literature et d'hisoire anciennes 1 (1845): 415-38

Stephen of Athens	6th to 7 C CE; physiological prccesses of urine formation; see Lucinan Rita Angeletti and Berenice Cavarra, "The Peri Ouron Treatise of Stephanus of Athens: Byzantine Uroscopy of the 6th-7th Centuries AD," American Journal of Nephrology 17 (1997): 228-32; In the 6th-7th centuries CE, treatises on uroscopy were written by Theophilus, Magnus and the author of work transmitted through the ms. Parisinus gr. 2260, Stephanus of Athens
Rhazes (865-925 CE)	A musician turned physician
Avicenna (980-1037 CE)	Work describining urine foreshadowed the science of uroscopy. One of Avicenna's renal advice advised uretheral insertion of a louse to improve urination

Theophilus	Byzantium 7th-9th C CE?; monographs on uroscopy; described twenty colors of urine; in 11th C uroscopic tracate translated and incorporated in *Articella* that emerged at the Salerno school; W Wolska Conus, "Stephanos d'athenes (d'Alexandrie) et Theophilie de Protospathaire, commentateurs des Aphorismes d'Hippocrates, sont-ils independants l'un de l'autre?" Revue des etudes byzantines 52 (1994): 5-58
Tibet Medical Treatise	See text rGyud bzhi; Influence of Arabic and Persian disseminator of Byantine uroscopic lore reached Tibet; see Ronit Yoeli-Tlalim, "On Urine Analysis and Tibetan Medicine's Connections with the West," in Studies of Medical Pluralism in Tibetan History and Society, ed. Sienna Craig, Minghi Cuomu, Frances Garrett, and Mona Schrempf, Beitrage zur Zentralaisenforschung 18 (Halle: International Institute for Tibetan and Buddhist Studies, 2010), 195-211
Isaac Israeli	North Africa, 9th C CE; Kitab al-bawl (Book of Urine);

Maimonides (1135-1204)	1134-1204; ch.5 of Medical Aphrorisms [on nephrology] in a series of excerpts mainly from Galen's commentary on Aphorisms 7:31-35 as well as Galen's De crisibus 1.12 etc.; Notes that he never witnessed anyone who urinated black urine survive.
Constantinus Africanus	Italy, 11th C CE; translated kitab al-bawl; see Eugenio Fontana, Il libro delle urine di Isacco L'ebreo, tradotto dall'arabo in Latino da Constantino Africano (Pisa: Casa Editrice Giardini, 1966)
Ibn Zarbala's	12th C CE Iberian Peninsula; sefer Sha'shu'im

Shlomo ben Abin

The Colors of Urine last quarter of 12th C Northern France ; four basic temparments: sanguinic, choleric, phlegmatic, and melancholic and four corresponding elementary qualities: cold, hot, dry, and humid. White urine= cold; red urine= hot; thick urine= humid; thin urine= dry; Red & thick= hot and humid= blood; Red & thin= hot and dry= red bile; white & thick= cold and humid= phlegm; White and thin= cold and dry= black bile; the origin of this semantic color code may be a section of Muhammad b. Zakariyya al-Razi (854-925) who wrote the medical compendium Kitab al Hawi translated in Latin as being authored by chamec filius tayp (Ahmad ibn al-Tayyib al-Sarakhsi in Baghdad; this taxonomy of signs are observable in the urine' Shlomo ben Abin explains red and thin urines as:

"בראותך השתן אדום ודק בלי עבות ובלי עכר תדון כי חליו מן המרה האדומה והיא קולרא רוביא האדם זהו הדם (צ'ל החם) והדקות הוא היובש וכן המרא האדומה חמה ויבשה ותדון בו חלי הראש עם קדחת שלישית או שאחזתו חמה וכאב הלב ועצירה וחולי המתנים והברכים ויובש הכבד וצמא ברוב חזה אז תשמרנו מכל דבר המחמם ותסוק בו בכל דבר המקרר ומלחלח כמו שאודי'ער במקומם"

(When you see that the urine is red and thin without thickness and murk, conclude that his diseases are due to red bile, which is cholera rubea. The redness is heat, and the thinness is dryness, and thus the red bile is hot, and dry. And you can conclude that the has diseases of the head with tertian fever, or that heat takes him and pain in the heart, and strangury, and disease of the hips, and the knees, and dryness of the liver.

Introduction 99

Doeg the Edomite

1197-1199 produced translations of urological texts from Latin into Hebrew; translated Articella; Hebrew translations of medical texts such as Hippocrats Aphorisms and works of Isaac Israeli and Theophilus

Mauro of Salerno

Italy, 12th C. CE; wrote tractate on Uroscopy (Regulae urinarum); vernacular uroscopic texts based on this; see Keil, "Die Urognostische Praxis," 136-41; Laurence Moulinier-Brogi, "La fortune du De urinis de Maurus de Salerne et ses volgarizzamenti inedits," Melanges de l'ecole Francaise der Rome, Moyen Age 122 (2010): 261-78; In *Regulae urinarum* we read, "שתן שוסיטירינא ועבה בכל בשוה קדחת קוטדיאנא מפלאמא נטוריל ויש לו כאב בחלצים ובראש ועצלות איבריו זרוק בפיו ובכול שעה מג' שעות ולמעלא מהלילה בקור ואחר כך מחמם " This can be compared in parallel Latin version in Regulae Urinarum Magistri Mauri in Collectio Salernitana,(ed Renzi 3:10): *Urina igitur in colore subcitrina, in substantia per totum et equaliter spissa sine lividitate, quotidianam significant de flegmate naturali. Ille ergo, vel illa, cujus est talis urina, quantum est in colore et substantia ipsius urine, nocte qualibet a teria ora noctis in antea predictis sinthomatibus debet infestari, primo frigore , deinde calore.*

Nathan ha-Meati

Translated Avicenna's Canon from Arabic to Hebrew and Hippocrates from Arabic to Hebrew ie. Aphorisms translated 1283 and Prognostics and Airs Waters Places. ; His son Shlomo ha-Meati translated Galen's commentary on the latter work from Arabic to Hebrew in 1299; The Hebrew medical lexicon includes: (a) mar'eh appearance; (2) annan (cloudy urine); (3) mayim muglim (water with pus); (4) mara aduma (red bile); consistency (mayim ie. Watery); (5) without fever בלא קדחת; (6) min (kind or genus), (7) mahloqet (division ie. Species); (8) a sign of ל את (8) on top of the urine (within the urine flask on top) מרום השתן (9) במרום השתן ברום השתן pain of the kidneys כאב הכליות (10) essence (ikar); (11) like the color of saffron (כמראה הכורבום) , (12) appearance of pale thin urine (panim mekhurkamot; The root krkm in Nitpa'el in Genesis Rabbah (parasha 99) means in the sense to "become pale" (13) natural phlegm ((;(כלאמא נטוריל (14) drops of blood in urine שתן בו כמראה כטפות דם

Gilles of Corbeil	Northern France, 13th C CE; urological treatise in form of didactic poem; see Aegidius Corboliensis (Gilles of Corbeil), Carmina medica, ed., Ludovicus Choulant (Leipzig: Leopold Voss, 1826)
William the Englishman	13th C CE challenge traditional Uroscopy ; see Moulinier-Brogi, Guillaume L'anglais le frondeur de l'uroscopie medieval, Edition commentee et traduction du De urina non vis (Geneve: Droz, 2011)
Johannes Zacharias Actuarius	14th C CE ca 1330 Byzantine monography on uroscopy; see
Morgagni (Giovanni Battista Morgagni) 1682-1771	Described various renal disorders via autopsy
Paracelsus (Theophrastus Bombastus von Hohenheim) 1493-1541); Switzerland	16th C CE; see Camille Viellard, *L'urologie et les medicins urologues dans la medecin ancienne* (Paris: FR de Rudeval, 1903), p. 99-103; wrote about proteinuria, hematuria, gout, and edema; forerunner of concept of specific gravity of urinalysis
Andreas Vesalius (1514-1564); born in Brussels	Father of modern anatomy; illustrated renal anatomy in his work De Humani Corporis Fabrica (1543)

Marcello Malphighi (1628-1694)	Identified the glomerulus (Malphigian corpuscle) and in 1666 published his observations on the kidney in De viscerum structura exercitation anatomica. He wrote of the pyramids of the renal medulla and collecting ducts as well as other microscopic aspects of the kidney; employed dye injection to describe glomeruli as "hanging like apples from the blood vessels, which when swollen with black fluid look like a beautiful tree"
Tovia Cohen (1652-1729)	1652-1729 Maaseh Toviah examines uroscopy, kidney function, body fluid homeostasis, obstructive uropathy (lived in Cracow, Naples, Adrinopole, Constantinople, buried in Jerusalem
Bartholomaeus de Montagnano (?-1460)	d. 1616 buried in Amsterdam; Painting attributed to Gerrit Dou (17th C) represents Jewish physician (probably Bartholemaeus) examining a flask of urine i.e. uroscopy
Lorenzo Bellini (1748-1795) Italy	*Exercitatio Anatomica de Structura Usu Renum* (1662)
Alexander Schumlanksy (1748-1795 Russia	De Structura renum (1782)

Modern History of Nephrology

On May 18, 2016 a nutshell posting of the brief history of nephrology was made online[79]

The text succinctly reads:

"The initial recognition of kidney disease as independent from other medical conditions is widely attributed to Richard Bright's 1827 book "Reports of Medical Cases," which detailed the features and consequences of kidney disease. For the next 100 years or so, the term "Bright's disease" was used to refer to any type of kidney disease. Bright's findings led to the widespread practice of testing urine for protein — one of the first diagnostic tests in medicine.

The study of kidney disease was furthered by William Howship Dickinson's description of acute nephritis in 1875 and Frederick Akbar Mahomed's discovery of the link between kidney disease and hypertension in the 1870s. Mahomed's original sphygmograph, created when he was a medical student, was improved in 1896 by Scipione Riva-Rocci, of Italy, with the use of a cuff to encircle the arm.

In the twentieth century, investigators such as Homer Smith revealed the underlying physiology of the kidney. Smith's findings led to

[79] web address: https://resident360.nejm.org/content_items/ 419 (NEJM Resident 360)

important medical therapies for multiple kidney diseases. As technology improved, therapy in the field of nephrology was further advanced with the first successful use of hemodialysis in 1945 by Willem Kolff. Shortly thereafter, in 1954, the first successful kidney transplantation was performed in identical twins in Boston by Joseph E. Murray. With further work in immunology, Murray and his team were later able to transplant kidneys into unrelated recipients with the use of immunosuppressive therapy. One of the first successful case series describing the use of immunosuppression (azathioprine or 6-mercaptopurine and glucocorticoids) was reported in the New England Journal of Medicine in 1963 by Murray and colleagues.

Today, clinical nephrology continues to advance with many forms of renal replacement therapy — both acute and chronic — including hemodialysis, peritoneal dialysis, hemofiltration and hemo diafiltration, the use of erythropoietin for anemia in chronic kidney ther disease, treatment of renal osteodystrophy, ongoing improvements in immunosuppression for transplantation, and specific treatments for many nephropathies."

This concise summary obviously does not contain details of the complicated development of modern nephrology from let us say the 17th century to the present. Below is a thumbnail sketch in the form of a timeline citing dates and names during this period significant to developments in modern nephrology as a discipline.

Time Line

1733 **Stephen Hally** – measure blood pressure in horse

1688 **Leonhard Thurneysser** – uroscopy, Basal Switzerland and Berlin, Was a goldsmith, miner, printer, uroscopist; introduced physicochemical methods into uroscropy. He proposed that urine distillates and their residues should be burnt in order to define their composition from the colour of the flame. He developed a theory of fractionated distillations

Richard Bright 1789-1858, (1) his work led to the recognition that coagulable protein in the urine indicates macroscopic kidney disease, (2) use of light microscopy introduced by Simon, Nasse, Henle, and Frerichs that helped identify constituents of urinary sediment. Becquerel described dysmorphic erythrocytes and Simon and Henle observed casts in urine and the histological preparations. Bird mentioned casts in passing but published the first book in urinary microscopy which allowed Bright in part to make his revolutionary contributions (3) While dropsy referred to symptoms perceived by the patient as well as the physician, Bright's disease focused mainly on microscopic pathology invisible to the patient, (4) in 1827 Bright provided the first almost complete clinical descriptions of the various forms of acute and chronic glomerulonephritis and showed that they were accompanied by macroscopic changes in the kidneys. (5) the finding of albuminuria with edemia meant the patient had renal disease. Between 1850 and 1885 Frerichs,

Klebs, and Langhands described primary glomeruclar lessions; In 1820 with Thomas Addison and Thomas Hodgkin formed Guy's Hospital; with Thomas Addison (1793-1860) and Thomas Hodgkins (1798-1866) one of the triumvirates of the London's Guy's Hospital. The medical research unit in his hospital provided descriptions of acute nephritus, nephrotic syndrome, uremia, small and enlarged kidneys, and the link between renal disease and enlarged ventricals of the heart; Bright made advances in neurology also such as Jacksonian seizures, infantile seizures, sringomyelia, brain arteries, and narcolepsy. Bright's observations of renal disease are preserved in the Gordon Museum of London's Guy's Hospital.

Sir Robert Christison 1797-1882, of Edinburgh was one of the 3 pioneers of modern nephrology along with Bright and Rayer. Christison confirmed and extended Bright's work on the nature of the origins of albuminuria and dropsy, (2) showed that these states might be reversible, (3) suggested a relationship between acute nephritis, large and granular kidneys, (4) discovered the basis for understanding uremia while applying chemistry to the study of blood and urine in patients with renal disease, (5) described and quantified the anemia of renal failures, (6) made microscopic examinations of the kidney and urine, (7) described the syndrome of acute renal failure from intrinsic renal involvement in response to outside poisons; Christianson expanded the understanding of uremia and anemia in renal failure, discerendd albuminuria and edema might be reversible in some situations, offered detailed microscopic studies of urine as well as the kidney and linked some cases of acute renal failure to toxins or posions.

Pierre-Francois Olive Rayer 1793-1867, (1) devised a method for the scientific study of diseases effecting the kidneys and urinary tract. (2) assembled vibrant illustrations of a wide range of disorders of the kidney found in specimens obtained at autopsy represented in his classic *Atlas of the Kidney*, (3) His 2100 page treatise titled *Traite des Maladies des Reins et des Alterations de la Secretion urinaire*, integrated the results of his pathological anatomical studies with urinary biology and clinical observations written between 1837-1841 in 3 volumes . (4) Rayer and Vigla identified for the first time elements other than crystals in urine and contributed to the methodology of handling samples for microscopy. While Lister had developed complex multi glass lenses in the 1820s, in the 1830s clinical urinary microscopy was pioneered by Rayer and his pupils in Paris especially Vigla. In the late 1830s this spread to the UK and Germany in the 1840s with detailed descriptions and interpretations of cells and formed elements of the urinary sediment by Nasse, Henle, Robinson and Golding Bird. Classes in its uses were held by Donne in Paris; Rayer advanced not only nephrology but physiology, pathological anatomy, comparative pathology, medical chemistry, and parasitology

Mahomed 1872- relationship between high blood pressure and renal disease

Claude Bernard 1813-1878; French physiologist .
He accomplished experiments in physiology that
set the sage for sound scientific methodology and is
acclaimed as father of modern physiology;
emphasized blind eperiments to ensure scientific
objectivity and he performed classic experiments
on the pancreas' function (discovered lipolytic
function of the exorcine pancreas) as well as the
glycogenic function of the liver with improvement
in knowledge of diabetes mellitus. First to describe
homeostatis or constancy of the internal
environment (le milieu interieur) and the
vasomotor system. Later in history principles of
perlustration to renal physiology i.e. 20th C
electrolyte content of le milieu interieur.

Theodor von Ferichs 1819-1885, performed
microscopic studies on Bright's disease and wrote a
textbook in German on nephrology titled, *Die
Brightsche Nierenkrankheit und deren Behandlung.*
Frerichs conducted clinical and microscopic studies
that led him to conclude that Bright's disease is a
single pathological entity with many causes. He
identified 3 stages through which the condition
progresses: (1) chronic renal disease, progresses to
end-stage renal failure with common features of
tubulointerstitial fibrosis and tubular atrophy.
Frerichs is better known for his contributions to
hepatology

William Griesinger 1817-1868; suggested in 1859
that diabetes might be causing Bright's disease,
with the later as a complication. This had
consequences for the next half century the
observation that as albuminuria appeared and
increased, so glycosuria improved or might remit,

with a parallel of subsequent evolution into uraemia.

Ludwig Traube (1818 in Ratibor, Silesia now Racibórz, Poland –1876 Berlin), (1) recognition of the pressure-volume relationship of urine output, (2) linked left ventricular hypertrophy with renal disease, (3) recognized that hypertrophy maintains circulatory homeostasis at a higher level of pressure; Traube considered the possibility of cardiac and renal disease could be the consequences of the same unknown disease, but rejected hypertrophy per se as a causal factor

Louis Pasteur 1822-1895; rabbies vacination and pasteurization process, germ theory

Gluge- first to see inflamed Malpighian bodies of the glomeruli although primary site of damage disputed by Henle, Pfeufer, Virchow, Reinhardt, and Frerichs

1873-1927 **Sergey Zimmicki**—Byelorussian physician, - founder of the urine concentration test 1866-1944 Sandar Korany, Hungarian scientist who described hyposthenuria in chronic renal failure

1872-1950 **Franz Vollhard** classified Kidney disease and with Fahr published classic on Bright's disease in 1914; Patients with chronic renal disease were advised to go to Assuan in Egypt where the warm sunny weather and low humidity were thought to decrease their urinary output.

J Roguski in Poznan continued research on water-electrolyte balance, metabolic and endocrine disturbances in renal patients and immunology of glomerular diseases. The first HD treatment was performed in Poznan in 1958 by the group of Roguski and coworkers chaired by K Baczyke

1898 **Tigerstedt and Berg** – relationship to renin and possible link to renal disease

Jakov Henle 1809–1885); The improvements in light microscopy allowed Henle to achieve advances in knowledge of the kidney. Particularly the advent of achromatic lenses made possible for Henle and his friend Schwann to uncover the typical structure of cells bringing a principle to the concept of living tissues. He argued that there are 4 basic types of tissue: (1) epithelial, (2) connective, (3) muscular, and (4) nervous in contrast to Bichat's 21 different types of tissues of different combinations in forming the organs of the body. Henle also observed micro-organisms in the excretions of diseased animals. He suggested this although he was unable to prove that microorganisms can cause disease. His discovery of the renal tubule now bears his name came relatively late in his career.

Carl Ludwig 1816-1895; arguments for hemodynamic physical forces mediated glomerular filtration

Hermann Senator December 6, 1834 – July 14, 1911 , by 1896 Senator had deduced that hyaline cylinders arise in the kidney tubules, (2) gave a classification of nephritis after term glomerulonephritis was coined by Klebs; (3) his observations of physiological and pathological protein excretion in humans became important; His investigations on urinary albumin excretion in individuals without primary kidney disease proved significant. He tried to disprove the held dogma that albuminuria was always a sign of primary renal disease. Today testing urinary albumin concentration by immune detection methods, as low level albumin excretion has turned out to be a predictor of cardiovascular and renal risk in diabetic and non diabetic patients which owes an early legacy to Senator.

William Bowman 1816-1892; moved along knowledge of renal structure and function notably the demonstration of the continuity of the glomerural capsule with the tubular basement membrane. He described the capsule around the glomerulus and gave his name to this part of the kidney

William Senhouse Kirkes 1822-1864; Ludwig Traub credits William Senhouse Kirkes for the key role for raised intra-arterial pressure as a pathogenetic agent in hypertension. Kirkes main interst was cardiology and vascular disease and gave the first account of embolism from vegetations in infective endocarditis in 1952. Three years later he published a study of apoplexy in Bright's disease, in which he notes clearly the role of raised intra-arterial tension in the causation of arterial disease. The inference of the existence of high blood pressure as a cause of renal disease in the mid 19th century evolved from Toynbee who noted medial hypertrophy and intimal narrowing of blood vessels in the kidney, while Johnson thought that kidney disease was the cause of compressed vessels. Johnson proposed a causal relationship between contraction of vessels and hypertrophy but never went beyond the insights articulated by Bright. Gull and Sutton disagreed with Johnson and proposed the presence of a general disease which leads to both cardiac hypertension and renal disease. It was Ewald in Germany who was able to ascribe both cardiac and vascular hypetrophy to increasing tension in the arterial system and one of the first to articulate the effect of hypertension on the kidney

Rudof Heidenheim 1834-1897; active tubular transport

Francis Delafield 1841-1915 (London, Berlin, NY); gave accurate microscopic descriptions of kidney pathology, made efforts to correlate clinical signs and symptoms with kidney lessions and provided a nosological classification of the acute and chronic forms of what was known then as Bright's disease; Graduated in 1963 from NY College of Physicians and Surgeons and continued studies in London and Berlin. Pioneer in renal histology correlating renal symptoms with kidney histological pathology. His work helped the later work of Segalas and Wohler on extra load of urea leading to diuresis, Ludwig's studies on urine fluctuations due to hypertension, Ustimowitch (with Falk and Richet) work on urinary solutes and renal flow, Cushney's work on what was later called osmotic diuresis, Friedrich von Mullers work on what he termed nophrosis in 1905 (vs. nephritus) etc.

Thomas Addis 1881-1949, Born in Scotland and trained in Edinburgh, he came to San Francisco in

1911 and moved forward knowledge of renal physiology, kidney disease, and body fluids in American Medicine, along with Donald D Van Slyke, John Peters, Homer W Smith, and Alfred Newton Richards. This group especially Homer Smith shaped interest in metabolic problems and pathophysiology. Thus acute renal failure emerged during WWII and fostered interest in hemodialysis and renal biopsy. Addis investigated the structure and function of the kidneys in Bright's disease, and studied kidney growth, hypertrophy and protein metabolism. Addis used the concept of Clearance as a measure of kidney function and was the first to systematize examinations of the urinary sediment-known as the Addis count. He also contributed to knowledge of diet and rest in treatment of Bright's disease. Addis's book, *Glomerular Nephritis: Diagnosis and Treatment,* is a classic of the field. He anticipated the trend to follow patients throughout their lifelong diseases thus trending theories of continuum of care and therapeutic alliance between patients and physicians. He also tailored prescriptions and frequency of controls to each individual patient and phase of the disease prescribing what was best for each case, thus anticipating tailored therapies; born and trained in Scotland but moved his research in 1911 to Stanford School of Medicine, recruited by Stanford's dean of medicine, Ray Lyman Wilbur. Named "Addis count of urinary sediment." Contributed to protein metabolism and renal growth (hypertrophy) and use of diet as well as rest in management of renal disorder. Studied blood coagulation and haemophilia research that included transfusing fresh blood into a patient with hemophilia to shorten the clotting time.

Homer W Smith, 1895-1962; Chair of Physiology at the Univ of Virginia but moved to NY University in 1928. Important work in glomerular filtration, tubular absorption, secretion of solutes in renal physiology. Established that the kidney worked according to principles in physiology both as a filter and a secretory organ. Removed the belief in vitalism in renal physiology that life's processes are not subject to laws of physics and chemistry alone. Spent many summers researching in Maine osteichthyes which led to his book *Fish to Philosopher. And Man and His gods* which has an introduction by Albert Einstein. Also authored book in 1951 that treated the pediatric kidney. Traced ontology of the kidney from fetal development to children to adults and maturation of renal function in childhood to adulthood by examination of relation of urine flow to filtration rate; urea clearace; maintenance of salt and water balance in infancy etc.

Alfred Newton Richards 1876-1966; Born in Stamford NY Richards was an important pharmacologist involved in the discovery of the mechanism of urine formation. He led a group of scientists at the Univ of Pennysylvania that meticulously established the physicology of renal glomerular filtration and selective tabular reabsorption.

Donald Dexter Van Slyke 1883-1971; Provided key concepts for scientists and clinicians on cardinal concepts of acid base balance. Allowed clinicians to more accurately understand diabetes and nephritus with particularly reference to acidosis and alkalosis. In 1918 published paper on lung volume and later a work on amino acids and the significance of the urea clearance in renal disease from the Rockefeller Institute for Medical Research in NY. This Dutch American Biochemist was a graduate of the Univ of Michegan; Developed field of quantative modern blood chemistry that included work on the measurement of gas and electrolytic levels in tissues. Co-authored Quantitative Clinical Chemistry with pioneer John P Peters

John P Peters (1887-1955); MD from Columbia College of Physicians and Surgeons and completed residency at Cornell Medical College. Worked at Rockefeller with Donald D Van Slyke and others in biochemistry before medical career at Yale University School of Medicine. His research aimed at improving knowledge to details of chemical make up of blood and urine as well as how these states were disrupted by renal diseases as well as other disorders (liver disease, diabetes mellitus etc) He applied principles of chemistry and physiology to his work including: the Starling law, the Donnan effect, the Henderson Hasselbalch equilibrium. Established the importance of the flame photometer to accurately measure sodium and potassium concentrations in small amounts of serum or urine, utilized the balance technique in clinical research, and able to integrate raw research data into clinical applications of patients with severe renal disease. Clarified areas such as Water balance in health and disease. Taught courses in metabolism, electrolyte and acid base equilibriums, nephritus, and water exchange. Cofounded field of quantitative clinical chemistry with Van Slyke.. His students include Robert Petersdorf, Lawrence R. Freedman, Jack Orloff, Arnold S. Relman, Franklin H Epstein, Donald Seldin, and others.

Thomas Graham 20 December 1805 – 16 September 1869; in 1861 found that colloid and crystalloid substances contained in fluids could be separated by diffusion of crystalloids through vegetable parchment acting as a semipermeable membrane. He coined the term dialysis

Jan Brod 1912-1985- Czech nephrologist developed clinical nephrology and renal replacement therapy

1934 **Goldblatt** renal hypertension produced by experiment which led to the elimination of the role of the kidney in human hypertension by a wide variety of methods

1935 **Paul Kimmelstiel and Clifford Wilson** 1935 paper; paper detailed nodular renal lesions in just 8 maturity-onset (48-68 year old) diabetics

1940s electron microscopes followed by the detection of specific proteins and cells using immunofluroescent antibodies

1941 **Arthur Allen,** clarified the association in 105 patients with diabetes over 40 years of age with kidney problems, confirming diabetic nephropathy as a disease. In the 1950s the technique of renal biopsy was applied to the study of diabetics and the early lessions defined using electron microscopy as well as sophisticated optical methods

Abel (Balto.) 1st dialysis of dogs with vivi diffusion (named Artificial Kidney

Haas (Germany) 1924 treated first time uremia in man with dialysis using colladian membrane and new ATG: "heparin." Gave up trials in 1928 with problematic results

Nils Aswal (Sweden); performed the first systematic aspiration needle biopsies of the kidney in 1944 but did not publish his results because of an early passing which led **him to abandon the technique.**

1951 Iveren and Brun (Copenhagen); when Iversen and Brun in Copenhagen described Aswal's results in 1951 a number of physicians around the world began to attempt renal biopsy using cutting and aspiration techniques.

Robert Kark (Chicago); developed renal biopsy to be more safe. Employed techniques of immunoflurorescence and electron microscopy

William Kolff (Netherlands)- built rotating drum kidney using cellophane and dialysis membrane. In the 1945 Kolff reported the first recovery of a patient undergoing HD for acute renal failure (ARF)

Societe de Pathologie Renale (France, Belgium, Switzerland), assembled just after WWII; first studies were physiopathological and bore on acute uremia and the associated hydromineral disorders, nephrotic syndromes, and the kidney of heart failure. Medical intensive care for kidney disease was developed and targeted on the hydromineral equilibrium.

1960, **Scribner and Quinton**- Teflon tubing; 1960 designed an external arteriovenous by pass made of Teflon tubing whih allowed permanent access to the bloodstream without the use of a permanent anticoagulation

Jean Hamburger, President of International Congress of Nephrology (Geneva) 1960 who reported and discussed at the 1st International Congress of Nephrology in Evian and Geneva progress in HD

Priscilla Kincaid Smith (1926-2015)- An Austrialia based South African physician and researcher who improved diagnosis and treatment of flomerulonephritis. In the 1960s she demonstrated evidence of links between headache powders containing phenoacetin and kidney cancer. Her research also showed connections between high blood pressure and renal malfunction. She was president of the Royal Australasian College of Physicians (1986-88). She was the director of Nephrology at the Royal Melbourne Hosptial (1967-91), Professor of Medicine (Univ. Of Melbourne 1975-91), Royal Physicican in Neprhology at Royal Womens' Hospital in Melbourne (1976-91).

Detective Sleuthing

Reconstructing the history of nephrology requires much detective work and sleuthing and interest on the part of the researcher, who must evaluate information on diseases of the kidney in various medical texts of the past, where it has sometimes been buried for centuries. We can often diagnosis *apres la lettre* that notable figures such as Samuel Johnson, Mozart, Beethoven, Disraeli, Brunel, and more recently Jean Harlow who suffered from symptoms of uraemia, passed on from renal failure if then unrecognized. In their day and age there was much more consciousness of maladies such as dropsy, with which renal disease had long been identified, but this was confused with the majority of cases of dropsy arising from heart failure and from liver disease. Cameron writes, "thus it is impossible to know from what condition the hydropic woman in Gerard Dou's famous painting in the Louvre may be suffering from. This was changed only when Richard Bright established the connection between dropsy with albumin in the urine and renal alterations in the 1820s and 1830s, which changed the name of the condition for the next century to Bright's disease, and introduced the idea of eponymy to medicine" (3-4).

During the Industrial Revolution in England it is estimated that chronic renal failure was 10x more common than today. According to Stewart Cameron in his book *A History of Treatment of Renal Failure by Dialysis* (Oxford: Oxford University Press, 2002), "This remained the case until the early years of the last century, up to the First World War, just as it remains in the developing world at the end of the twentieth century." Acute and chronic renal failure were then reframed rather abruptly around 1950-1960 by the introduction of dialysis. This history is addressed in G. Richet's *Histoire de l'hemodialyse dans l'uremie aigue* in *Review Praticien,* 1992. Further the work, *The development of hemodialysis and peritoneal dialysis* edited by A.R. Nissenson, R.N Fine, and D.E. Gentile has appeared in its 3rd edition with Prentice Hall International (London, 1995).

Today haemodialysis represents the successful application of physical chemistry and physiology, together with materials and mechanical science to a pressing clinical problem. E Capodicasa and M. Timio in their article "When the history of nephrology changed that of medicine" (G. Ital Nefrol, 2004, May-June 21 (3) 254-8) argue that six milestones have marked the medical and scientific human progress which are: (1) Galen, the ligature of the ureters and the birth of experimental medicine, (2) uroscopy and introduction of laboratory exams, (3) the synthesis of urea in the laboratory and the beginnings of biotechnology, (4) the kidney and the introduction of systematic parenteral antibiotic therapy, (5) the kidney and the first artificial organs, (6) the kidney and the start of the transplantation era. This sixfold development should also incorporate the role of chemistry and cell biology for modern nephrology which requires a background in bio-chemistry. Chemistry evolved from a descriptive to an analytical, organic, biological, and physical science that replaced animism with physiochemical forces and laws of chemical reactions that govern matters of life. Cell biology on the other hand established the cell as the structural and functional unit of living organisms. Refined microscopic technologies then helped to identify the structural components of the cell in greater detail amongst which the plasma membrane was of key importance in regulating the separation of the intracellular machinery from its environment and thereby maintaining a balance of harmonious cell relationships. The interaction of chemistry and cell biology led to the establishment of better understanding the role of renal tubules in the vital function of the kidney in maintaining body homeostasis.

Renal Imaging techniques have advanced from the past to today so that while the ancients relied on the naked eye in often forbidden dissection we have seen the evolution of micro dissection and maceration of silicone rubber injected tubules. Imaging evolved from naked eye observation to magnifying lenses, microscopes and finally electron microscopy. This allowed focus on the site of urine formation, and inspection of renal structures in the renal medulla and the imaging of tight junction strands, by non invasive techniques such as X ray imaging, imaging by radioisotopes, ultrasound computer tomography and nuclear magnetic resonance. Micropuncture and microperfusion techniques have opened the field for direct imaging not only for renal details but also the functional parameters such as transtubular reabsorption rates, single glomerular capillary filtration and conductance of the paracellular pathway.

As science advances and perfects potential survival on haemodialysis has been remarkable. The science of dialysis is based in part on the processes of osmosis, diffusion, and semipermeable membranes. The development of anti-coagulation and extra corporeal circuits helped the development of haemodialysis. The discovery and search for better membranes such as the peritoneum led to peritoneal dialysis. The first haemodialyses in humans was also possible by the use of hepearin and cellophane. The first practical dialysis machines for filtering the blood from uraemic toxins was made by Kolff, Murray, and Alwall. The invention of the flame photometer required urologists and nephrologists to work together more closely. The designs of the artificial kidney also represent a significant development.

The availability of new biological and synthetic materials in permitting the science of dialysis to be applied to the clinal problems of kidney failure including dialysis membranes, anticoagulants, and plastic polymers has made great advances in increasing longevity. The work of Kolff during WWII in the Netherlands has been noted.

Transplantation today provides a safe outlet for number of mostly younger patients.

Amyloidosis has not been the only new plague for the dialysis patient- other blood borne viruses such as hepatitis C are now recognized to be more dangerous than hepatitis B, and the unforeseen pandemic of AIDS beginning in the early 1980s has put dialysis at risk. This is due primarily to the dependence on blood access for dialysis treatment. Today the obesity crisis is also leading to higher instances of diabetes that can lead to end stage renal failure.

Politically much awaits to be worked out between the Scylla and Chrybdis of socialized medicine and privatization so that dialysis become available more easily in its fiscal and socio-economic context. Bio-ethicists are required to deal with the complicated dynamics of who should be recipients of organ donations or whether everything should be based on triage? Sometimes costs versus quality of life issues are considered.[80] Perhaps Jewish law with the ethical halakhic concerns is best sensitive to examine this complicated area of fairness, equity, and rights to health care with regard to organ donation and living donars.[81] If the business of "harvesting organs for donation" operates along economic models then human dignity and ethical breaches can arise in Jewish law that alerts us to the moral risks of the complications regarding organ donation.[82]

The role of women in nephrology is also a positive change in the signs of the times. While the medieval women Tratula wrote an important work in gynecology to Florence Nightingale (1823-1910) who organized women into the professional field of nursing to the first modern women to take her degree in medicine named Elisabeth Blackwell who

[80] Rozenbaum, E.A., Comparative study of costs and quality of life of chronic ambulatory peritoneal dialysis and hemodialysis patients in Israel / E.A. Rozenbaum [et al.]., Israel Journal of Medical Sciences 21,4 (1985) 335-339

[81] See Flaum, Tzvi, Living donor organ transplants, Medicine and Jewish Law III (2005) 131-140; Halperin, Mordechai, Organ transplants from living donors, Assia - Jewish Medical Ethics 2,1 (1991) 29-37; Rabinovitch, Nachum L, What is the Halakha for organ transplants?, Tradition 9,4 (1968) 20-27.

[82] Al, Joop, Comparative observations on some current medico-legal issues in Dutch law, Jewish Law Annual 12 (1997) 167-215

graduated from the Geneva Medical School of Western New York in 1849, the role of women continues to increase in medicine which is a good thing. Many thousands of books in the area of Women and medicine and science have arisen including: Margaret Rossiter's *Women Scientists in America*, (JHU Press, 1995), Wendy Williams's *Why aren't More Women in Science* (APA,2007) Laura Kelly's *Irish Women in Medicine* c. 1880s -1920s (Manchester, 2015), Majorie Bowman's *Women in Medicine* (NY: Springer, 2002), *Women in Medicine: an Encyclopedia* (Sage, 2002)., Carolyn Skinner's *women physicians in 19th C America* (Southern Ill Univ. Press, 2014), Ann Boulis' *Changing Face of Medicine* (ILR Press, 2008), etc.[83] However Harry Friedenwald in his monumental set *The Jews and medicine* in his chapter (XIII) titled 'Jewish Doctoresses in the Middle Ages" which first appeared in *The Medical Pickwick* (vol 6, Aug, 1920) shows that Jewish women have always been involved in the art of healing.

In 2002 an important work appeared based on a conference on the History of Nephrology, at the 3rd Congress of the International Association for the History of Nephrology, Taormina, November 2001: Reports. The blurb on the book states:

"Reconstructing the history of nephrology is not an easy task: It requires a great deal of

---

[83] *Bold Women of Medicine* by Susan Latta, 21 Stories of Astounding Discoveries, Daring Surgeries, and Healing Breakthroughts (2017), *Women Physicians and Cultures of Medicine* ed. Ellen S. More et. al., Baltimore: JHU Press (2009).

effort and interest on the part of the researcher, who has to explore information on diseases of the kidney in various medical texts of the past, where it has sometimes been buried for centuries.

This volume of 'History of Nephrology' thus concentrates on the history of diseases of the kidney. Physicians have toiled in diagnosing and treating ailments of the kidney for millennia, well before the emergence of the specialty of nephrology. It is also evident that many of the best minds in medicine, when faced with the complex signs and symptoms we now classify as diseases of the kidney, were initially puzzled by them and then satisfied by merely describing them. While the thriving of anatomy allowed some of these clinical manifestations to be attributed to pathologies of the kidney observed at autopsy, it was only after the Scientific Revolution and during the era of Enlightenment that most of these descriptive entities came to be grouped under the taxonomic terms by which any medical student today can make a specific diagnosis of kidney disease. Their treatment, however, whether symptomatic or curative, had to await the post World War II period of flourishing basic research. Nephrologists as well as those interested in the history of medicine in general will find this book a veritable treasure trove of information "

The Table of contents of Reprint of: American Journal of Nephrology 2002, Vol. 22, No. 2-3 can be found at https://www.karger.com/Journal/Issue/227786

This volume was preceeded in 1966 with History of Nephrology 2: Reports from the First Congress on the International Association for the History of Nephrology, Kos, October 1996. by Garabed Eknoyan (Author, Editor), Spyros G. Marketos (Editor), Natale Gaspare De Santo (Editor), Shaul G. Massry (Editor), N. G. De Santo (Editor)

In 2004 Dr Levy was asked to review a volume of this series which appeared with Oxford University press in *the Journal of the History of Medicine and Allied Sciences* volume 59, Number 3, Jully 2004 (E-ISSN: 1468-4373; Print ISSN: 0022-5045. See https://academic.oup.com/jhmas/article/59/3/481/749685

Dr. Levy's favorable review reads:[84]

History of Nephrology 4: Reports from the Third Congress of the International Association for the History of Nephrology
Garabed Eknoyan, Natale G. De Santo, Shaul M. Shasha, Guido Bellinghieri, Vincenzo Savica, Shaul G. Massry
Basel, Switzerland S. Karger AG
2002 vi, 218 illus. $64.50
cloth

---

[84] On 2/1/18 The Oxford Journal Permissions team gave permission to reprint this review (11:25 am)

To borrow a phase from Hippocrates: the life of nephrology as a speciality may be short, but its art is quite long, as is demonstrated by the recent fourth volume in the series History of Nephrology.

This book collects papers that were given at the Third Congress of the International Association for the History of Nephrology (IAHN) in October 2000. A picture of the conference site in Tyaorimina Sicily, beautifully reproduced on the cover, suggests at least one superficial attraction for its far-flung participants. The contributors represent a sampling of countries, including Bulgaria, France, Belgium, Greece, the United Kingdom, Israel, Italy and the United States.

The IAHN was founded in 1991, and the first session as held in Naples, Italy in October 1993. The proceedings of this and subsequent congresses appeared originally in *American Journal of Nephrology* and have been reproduced in separate volumes by its its publisher, S. Karger AG.

The current *History of Nephrology* 4 is a brilliantly formatted edition on high-quality, nonacidic paper with ample drawings and photographs, many in color. The publishers have a notable precedent. The original 1827 edition of Richard Bright's *Medical Cases Reports* employed the work of engraver Frederick R. Say, who relied on his day's high standard of mezzotint lithographs. Unlike Bright's book, however, which cost roughly ten times the prices of the average medical book of its day,
` 4 is reasonably priced and readily available.

Although there are many scattered articles on the history of nephrology in general textbooks and published articles, here are gathered reports by practicing nephrologists exploring the history of their own field. There is again, a notable precedent. Pierre Rayer, in the last hundred pages of his 1849 *Traite des Maladies des Reins*, received and critically evaluated the literature on nephrology from Hippocrates to his own time. *History of Nephrology* 4 examines selected aspects of this history to our present times and explores in detail both the ancient and more recent roots of this new specialty.

An introductory essay, "On the Continued Reconstruction of the History of Nephrology" by the editors states: "In helping reconstruct the history of diseases that constitute the matrix of nephrology, the IAHN has entered a new phase in its evolution.... [reconstructing] components of the edifice which constitutes the history of nephrology (p.2). There then follows several sections on the origins of nephrology in magic and myth, in antiquity, the Middle Ages, and the Renaissance. The modern era is covered with a review of the contribution of Harvey Lester White, R.F. Pitts, V. du Vigneaud, and John P. Peters. Also included is a section on the development of concepts of renal disease, such as acute and chronic renal failure, nephrotic syndrome, and immunology. Finally there is a section on therapeutics.

This format is a convenient way of organizing into workable sections these thirty-three various papers delivered at the Congress. In the future, I hope the authors would consider focusing on a major subject or a symposium on a defined topic, rather than arbitrarily arranging the diverse papers into set categories. In *the History of Nephrology* 3, such a symposium on the origins of renal physiology was presented with excellent results.

The last paper on the origins of nephrology is titled, "History of Nephrology in the Talmudic Corpus" by Dr. Estee Dvorjetski. At twenty-three pages it is the longest and most detailed article in the volume, with forty three well-chosen and pertinent references. Dvojetski shows that the Bible considered the kidneys symbols of the human emotions, contrary to the heart, which was regarded as the location of wisdom and understanding. Extensive evaluation of biblical and Talmudic literature is used to indicate the sages' concern with size of the kidney, presence of fluid or pus, and diseases such as urolithiasis, and urinary retention among others.

Another outstanding paper is by Gabriel Richet from Paris titled "Nephrolithiasis at the Turn of the 18th to 19th Centuries: Biochemical Disturbances." Richet comments that although kidney stones had been described since antiquity, the chemical analysis of stones in the late eighteenth century provided a firm basis for the developing field of chemistry. The author points out that Karl William Scheele in 1776, identified lithic acid (uric acid) as a component of urinary stones. W.H. Wollaston in England identified sodium urate in gouty deposits. Also identified in calculi were calcium phosphate and triple ammonium and magnesium phosphate. The studies of Fourcroy and Vauquelin as well as P. Rayer in France and Marcet and Prout in England helped apply chemical and clinical analysis using urinary calculi as a model for study. As the author indicates, these studies "established the place of chemistry in medicine and deeply contributed to the then budding discipline of metabolic physiology and pathology" (p.162).

History of Nephrology 4, as well as the preceding volumes, is recommended to those interested in the history of medicine and especially to nephrologists who desire to learn about the background of their specialty. It is a welcome addition to the history of medicine and nephrology.
DOI 10.1093/jhmas/jrh095
End of review

Chapter One

The Reception in Britain and on the Continent of Richard Bright's Reports of Medical Cases Linking Dropsy, Coagualable Urine and Small Granular Kidneys as a Clinical Entity—Edinburgh, Dublin and Paris

In 1827 Richard Bright from the Guy's Hospital in London published *Reports on Medical Cases selected with a view of Illustrating the Symptoms and Cure of Diseases by reference to Morbid Anatomy*. While the title doesn't refer to kidney disease or promote a cure, this book for the first time describes a clinical entity correlating the findings of dropsy or edema and coagulable urine with small granular kidneys. While Bright was not the first to make the observation that coagulable urine and dropsy could be related in certain patients, William Wells and John Blackall had made this observation, Richard Bright was the first to correlated these findings at autopsy with small granular kidneys, beautifully illustrated with lithographic prints. Heart failure, liver disease and tumors were ruled out as a cause of the dropsy.

Introduction

How quickly was the recognition and confirmation of Bright's findings made after this publication in 1827. Without the New York Times or the Wall Street Journal to promulgate medical discoveries, much less medical journals and frequent meetings to distribute new information, ideas and new discoveries circulated slowly in the early nineteenth century. Some discoveries are quickly taken up. Edward Jenner's report of vaccination was taken up by Napoleon who vaccinated his troops within several years. Clinically and pathologically renal diseases had been almost an unknown entity. However within ten years of Bright's publication the eponym *Morbus Brightii* or in France, *Maladie de Bright* was in common usage. While Bright's book has never been translated into German or French, in 1830 and 1832 brief reports of his findings appeared in the *Archive de Medecine*.

Comparison of the Publications of Bright, Christison and Rayer

Two volumes confirming and extending the findings of Bright were published, one in Scotland at Edinburgh by Sir Robert Christison, entitled *On Granular Degeneration of the Kidnies and its connection with dropsy, inflammation and other diseases* appeared in 1839 (the spelling kidnies is old Scots). This had been preceded in 1829 only two years after Bright's original publication by an article entitled *Observations on the the Variety of Dropsy which is Depends on Disease of the Kidney.* The other volume is by Pierre Rayer in Paris, an extensive two volume book including a massive Atlas, entitled *Traite des Maladies de Rein in 1840.* Sir Robert Christison had been several years behind Bright in medical school at Edinburgh and shared many of his teacher. His volume in 1839 was rather lean without engravings and directed primarily to the practitioners of the day. Pierre Rayer massive three volume set was comprehensive in scope, classifying various forms of renal disease with an atlas showing not only the granular shrunken or large pale kidneys as Bright had done but included malignacies, tuberculosis, calculi obstructing kidneys, etc. While a vast atlas, four by three and a half feet in size, the quality of the engraving doesn't come up to that in Richard Bright's volume in my opinion. Sir Robert gives credit to Dr Bright in the opening sentence of his preface, and praises his endeavors. Rayer does credit Bright with one of twelve categories of his break down of renal diseases-naming it Nephritie albumineuse . In the second volume of Rayer's book there are extensive references to Bright's work as well his circle of chemist – John Bostock, William Prout, and George Owen Rees, mainly in the extensive footnotes which represent a running dialogue to the body of the text. Except for the critical point of relating albuminuria with each of his cases, Bright paid little attention to the urine, although he described in detail the characteristics of the precipitate formed by the urine held in a spoon over a candle, further describing the urine as scanty of light coloured or dingy brown. He never reported examining urine under the microscope. Rayer on the other hand, recognizing the advancement of Charles Louis Chevalier who developed an achromatic lens allowing urine to be brought into focus under a microscope, studied the urine in this fashion and produced beautiful charts of casts, white cell, red cells, crystals of uric acid, cystine, phosphate of ammonia, oxalate, hipuric acid, and even crystals of quinine sulfate. Neither Bright nor Rayer examined tissue sections under the microscope; this would require knowledge of sectioning tissues with a microtome to make the sections thin enough for examination and further experience with achromatic lenses in the microscope.

Sir Robert Christison, Bart.

Robert Christison (1797-1882) led a long and productive life as a physician in Edinburgh. He was eight years younger than Richard Bright, who attended medical school at Edinburgh, but returned to Guy's Hospital in London. Christison is probably best known for his studies on poisonings and was twice President of the Royal College of Physicians and Professor of Medicine at Edinburgh. He has been called the Bright of Scotland on the basis of his book, *Granular degeneration of the Kidnies and its connection with dropsy, inflammation and other diseases*, published in 1839. His autobiography, edited by his sons and published in 1885, gives a detailed account of his interest and contribution to the acceptance of Bright's findings in Britain. To quote from Volume I, p382, "Very soon after the publication of Dr Bright's *Hospital Reports*, my attention was riveted on that portion of the work which announced his great discovery of the relation between dropsy and a previously unknown organic disease of the kidneys. I had written an analysis of that investigation for the *Medical and Surgical Journal* for July 1828; and at the same time I began to observe cases of the disease under my charge in the hospital." Christison goes on the indicate " that Bright's discoveries "were received at first with coldness by his brethren. It was said that such cases as he described had been seen only in Guy's Hospital, and in the scum alone of the London population." He goes on to state "The first confirmation of Bright's propositions proceeded from a paper published by me in the *Edinburgh Medical and Surgical Journal* for October 1829.The same incredulity attended at first my announcement of Bright's disease being prevalent in in Edinburgh. It was thought to occur in Infirmary practice alone, and only among the labouring community." Christison indicates further in his autobiography, "In a law action as to the nullity of a deed on the ground of its having been executed on deathbed, two physicians, one of them a lecturer on the practice of physic (medicine), had the audacity to swear in court that the testator could not have died of Bright's disease, as the chief witness for the prosecution suggested, because that disease was unknown in the middle ranks of life."

Indifference and Opposition to Bright's Findings among the Medical Profession

While Robert Christison accepted the findings of Richard Bright very promptly, his above statement that these ideas "were received at first with coldness by his breath and considered to be seen only at Guys Hospital in the scum alone of the London population" must be considered since all new ideas place a strain on accepted patterns of considering disease processes. Dropsie was considered a disease or more specifically an inflamation in itself, making appearances various parts of the body. Ascities was considered an inflamation of the abdomen and didn't require the kidneys to explain its etiology. James C. Gregory was a young colleague of Dr. Christison who contributed on his own to the acceptance of Bright's demonstrations, but in a paper, *On Diseased States of the Kidney connected during Life with Albuminous Urine* appearing in the London Medical Gazette of August 1831 confirms that, " I am not aware that any other physician in this country has turned his attention (other than Dr. Christison) particularly to the subject. The only public notice I have observed taken of the subject in this country has been by two distinguished clinical teacher, Dr. Elliotson of London and Dr. Graves of Dublin. By the reports of the lectures of these genelemen, it would seem that neither of them is satisfied as to the correctness of Dr. Bright's views regarding the supposed intimate connexion between organic disease of the kidney and coagulable urine.

Dr. John Elliotson was a distinguished physician and teacher at St. Thomas's Hospital and the University College London. His objection to coagulable urine indicating organic disease of the kidney was that most of his cases recovered and were restored to perfect health so that a functional congestion of the kidney rather than organic disease of the kidney was present. Gregory counters this argument by noting that that was not in accord with the results of the experience in the Edinburgh Infirmary. He grants that "urine becomes at times albumninous in certain peculiar states of the general system unconnected with organic alterations of structure in these organs. But when the urine is coagulable, and at the same time decidedly low in density, while it is below the natural standard in quantity, when this state of the urine has existed for some time in a more or less marked degree and when it is accompanied by dropsical effusion in some of its forms, or when in the absence of dropsy, which is by no means a constant symptom, it is attended by intractable vomiting or diarrhea...it is a sign of organic disease of the kidney on which we may rely with much confidence." Gregory grasp of the clinical condition of renal failure without laboratory tests so soon after Bright's original description is striking.

Nevertheless, Dr. Elliotson continued his opposition to acceptance to Bright's demonstration and in his lectures published as the opening article on Disease of the Urinary Organs in the London Gazette from August and September 1833, fails to mention Bright's name, discusses Nephritis (ie an inflammation of the Kidney) as representing a condition of pain in the loins and testicle, differentiating it from rheumatism. Alson discussed in this section is Diabetes, primarily considered as a kidney disease allowing sugar to appear in the urine (no acceptable blood determination for glucose had been forthcoming) and of course renal calculi. In his Principles and Practice of Medicine (a title cooped in 1892 by William Osler) of 1844, Elliotson gives Bright credit for having "collected a large number of cases, and he finds that when the kidney is in a disorganized state, the urine generally is albuminous." Then follows the disclaimer paragraph, *Organic Disease not Necessarily present*. The argument has not changed from that described by Dr. Gregory; "When the urine is albuminous, it does not follow that the kidney must be in a state of organic disease,etc." Dr. Elliotson certainly was not a true believer in the findings of Richard Bright as were Christison and Rayer.

The second physician mentioned by Dr. James Gregory as not being satisfied as to the correctness of Dr. Bright's views regarding the " supposed intimate connexion between organic disease of the kidney and coagulable urine was Dr. Robert Graves of Dublin, the Dr Graves most famous for his paper on *Newly Observed Affection of the Thyroid Gland in Females* in the London Med and Surg. Journal of 1835, describing hyperthyroidism. According to Gregory, Dr. Graves "considered that an albuminous state of the urine may occur in dropsies unconnected with disease of the kidneys. The occurrence of pale urine containing a small quantity of albumen and of unusually l9ow specific gravity indicating a diminution of the quantity of urea, may be considered characteristic of chronic hepatitis." Gregory goes on to explain why the liver is an unlikely cause of coagulable urine. He concludes, " from the cases published by Dr. Bright, as well as from daily experience, extensive alteration of structure is frequently found in the liver, without coagulability of the urine, if there is no concomitant disease of the kidneys." Dr. Elliotson concludes his paragraph on albuminous urine not necessarily representing organic kidney disease with a bow to Dr. Graves, "Dr. graves has done much t9o dissolve the supposed invariable connection between albuminous urine and disease of the kidney. He shows that it often depends on disease of the *liver"*, with a reference in a footnote or his valuable papers in the *Dublin Journal of Medical Science,*Vol.1.-11

A letter from Robert Graves to Richard Bright dated 31st December 1838 will give a flavor of the times and explain Graves' position:

Dear Sir

Your letter gave me much pleasure indeed, and that for several reasons- First, I rejoice at the opportunity of making an acquaintance by letter with me from whose writings I have derived so much instruction and profit-Secondly I still more rejoice at finding that we do not differ much if at all, concerning the connection between albuminous urine and structural disease of the kidney- I think you should do well to publish in the Medical Gazette a short expose of your opinions on the subject, for certainly your views have been very generally misunderstood both here and in America. <u>The matter is one of much practical importance for the idea is now too prevalent that abluminous urine invariably denotes in dropsy organic renal disease—I am much disposed to doubt</u> – but what use in repeating what I have printed—Let us break new ground- Can you, or can any of hour friends aid me in making a good map of the progress of the Indian Cholera-I want dates of its arrival at each important city or point of access- Such a map I know was published on the continent, but it was at an early period- I am much at a loss for data for America, Portugal, Spain and Italy – I believe Genieva and Switzerland generally escaped. Another pivotal point is to ascertain etc,etc on the logistics of the cholera epidemic, concluding, so if you can get me references or books where the information I seek is to be found, you will confer a very great obligation on me ----- Yours faithfully   Robert J Graves

The letter breaks off in the middle with what seem to be much more on Graves's mind, ie the Cholera epidemic rather than the fine points of albuminous urine and kidney disease.

Robert Christison's Efforts to Popularize and Extend Bright's Observations

Returning to Robert Christison who goes on to indicate "about this time, I was consulted in my first case in point (ie: a case of Bright's disease), that of an army officer; Dr. Abercrombie who very early saw the truth in his extensive practice; and by-and-by Bright's disease was recognized in all stations of life, by all medical men, and only in too great abundance." Dr Christison further indicates that his paper of 1829, describing seven cases of proteinuria and dropsy, only two years after Bright's original publication of 1827, and the first such paper to confirm Bright's results, "went avowedly no farther than to confirm, on a new field of observation, the main features and many details of Bright's admirable inquiry." He further indicates, "the only novelty of any consequence was a complete demonstration by chemical analysis of the occasional presence of urea in the blood - a fact which some experiments supplied to Bright by Dr. Bostock had obscurely indicated, and which seemed to be observable whenever the daily discharge of urea by the kidneys was materially defective."

In Bright's original 1827 publication of *Case Reports*, John Bostock is quoted in three letters, describing the urine and blood of three of Bright's cases. Specific Gravity, high albumin in dropsical urine and low value in the blood are described. Only in the second volume of *Cases and Observation of Bright in the Guy's Hospital Reports* of 1838, did Bostock report the presence of urea in hydrocephalic brain fluid in several patients who had seizures as part of their uremic syndrome. Bright in this 1838 ;publication gave credit to Doctor Robert Christison of Edinburgh for this demonstration of elevated urea in the blood of patients with renal disease. George Owen Rees in a later publication, On the Analysis of the Blood and Urine, 1848, details a meticulous and laborious method for the isolation of urea from the blood. We must accept Christison statement that the demonstration of elevated urea in the blood in renal disease was "a novelty of (some) consequence."

Christison's method of demonstrating urea in that 1829 report employed semi qualitative analysis using a crude extraction of blood with alcohol, filtering and drying and combining with Nitric Acid to produce crystals of the nitrate of urea, stating "these evidently were scales of nitrate of urea." William Cruikshank, Apothecary to the Army Hospital at Woolwich had been th4e first to isolate urea with Nitric Acid in 1798. This was recognized by Fourcroy in France, although he claimed priority in describing the method of isolation. Christison's isolation of the nitrate of urea was a qualitative, far from elegant chemical procedure, the end product of which consisted of "a considerable number of brown crystal scales having the odor of urine" By 1848, George Owen Rees, one of the animal chemists in the circle of Richard Bright, described an elegant, meticulous and laborious method for the isolation of urea using Nitric Acid that would be suitable for quantative analysis.

Another observation of Christison in his paper of 1829 was the potential reversibility of Brights's disease. All of Bright's patients died and had autopsies. As indicated by Christison " Another point of some consequence was an indication, fully established afterwards, that the disease is not the deadly, incurable malady pointed at by the experience of its first observer (ie; Richard Bright), but that it might be much mitigated, arrested in its progress, or even cured." Pierre Rayer's publication of *Traite des Maladies de Rein* in 1840 also recognized the potential reversibility of Bright's disease.

Christison's example of the potential reversibility of Bright's Disease is cited in Case 29 of his 31 case reports of 1839. The patient was named Mossman age 42, and as with Richard Bright, there is an indication of his occupation and mention of any substance abuse. The patient was a harbour porter, described with a " tall slender form, active, robust and long much addicted to intemperance" He was attacked February, 1836 with a violent inflammation of the left lung, probably pneumonia. Initially there was no proteinuria, but after one month the urine output decreased and coagulable urine and edema occurred. By the middle of April, now two months after admission he was improving; the urine protein was considerably reduced and " not long afterwards he went to the country to recovery his strength." No further follow up is available on Mr Mossman, but it may be assumed he is an example of acute renal failure with recovery. Actually Mr. Mossman was only one of twelve who recovered or went into remission so that they could be discharged from the hospital, among the thirty one patients described by Dr Christison in the 1839 publication of *Granular Degeration of the Kidnies*. The tabulation below will give a breakdown of the outcomes of Chrisitson's thirty one cases of what he calls granular degeneration:

Autopsy	17
No autopsy	2
Recover, no follow up	9
Remission with subsequent	2
death and no autopsy	
Remission with subsequent	
death and autopsy	1

	31

Since thirteen of the thirty-one patients described had no autopsy, it is possible that the granular degeneration diagnosed by Dr. Christison might not entirely fulfill the criteria of Richard Bright.

Robert Christison goes on to indicate that "Bright's disease proved to be so common in all ranks of society, that I had soon very ample opportunities for further observation; and consequently my materials relative to this subject accumulated, and appeared valuable enough to be produced in a separate work, which appeared in 1839 under the title of a treatise *On Granular Degeneration of the Kidneys'*. This volume is a realatively compact publication that consists of a Preface, thirty cases describing history, pathological findings, related diseases present, and discussion of causes, prognosis and treatment. No illustrations accompany this work , in comparison with the publications of Richard Bright and the subsequent publication of Pierre Rayer in 1838.

The preface of *On Granular Degeneration of the Kidneys'* and written in a lucid and charming style. The recognition of the priority of Richard Bright's publication is celebrated right up front in the very first paragraph. Christison. It is then noted that others previously had noted the presence of albuminuria in dropsy, ie: Blackwell, Wells, etc. Christison notes, "It was afterwards found, as in regard to many other important discoveries in pathology, that various authors had previously made observations which, if followed out, might have led them on to general principles established by Dr. Bright. It is not, however, by a few fortuitous observation, and still less by obscure and incomplete induction, that the merit of an original discovery in medical science is to be either gained on the one hand or lost on the other." He goes on in this preface to note that "Formerly, physicians were in possession of only a few scattered facts and dubious inferences respecting the connection between dropsy and diseased kidney, and there were almost disregarded, alike in science and in practice. Now they may become intimately acquainted with a disease of extreme frequency, which manifests itself by characteristic symptoms and singularly modifies and engenders a great variety of other long familiar maladie. For this important step in the progress of knowledge, medicine is indebted to Dr. Bright, - together with those enquires, whom his discovery has called forth, to explore with more minuteness the regions he has pointed out."

After this panegyric to Richard Bright, he addresses the problem as just why it has taken so long for the reluctant community to accept the findings of Richard Bright, which he, Robert Christison has embraced so promptly and enthusiastically embraced. "Not withstanding the novelty and interest of these researches, some time elapsed before they reached the attention which they ought at ours to have commanded. My position, as one of the physicians of the Infirmary of the City, having given me an opportunity of repeating and verifying the material parts of Dr. Bright's statements, I made the results public in a short paper in 1829. And in 1831 my late lamented friend and colleague in the hospital, Dr James Gregory, ably followed up and strengthened this confirmation by a comprehensive digest of his own experiences, as well as of that of myself and his other hospital colleagues, for the two proceeding years. Nevertheless, several years more passed by before the subject was taken up anywhere else, and to the present day strand as it may seem, Guy's Hospital in London and the Edinburgh Infirmery continue to be the only institutions of the kind in Britain which may be said to have contributed to the general stock, in the brand of pathological knowledge." To add a final volley of incredulity, Christison adds, " I found to my surprise, that by some medical gentleman of the metropolis the doctrines of Dr B. continue to be called into question."

He discusses further in the Preface what the condition should be called. He notes the Richard Bright did not name the disease. He objects to Pierre Rayer's designation Albuminous Nephritis (Nephrite Abumineuse), and comes to the astute conclusion that "further pathological research will probably show that there is more than one organic derangement" in the condition described by Bright.

Indeed pathological microscopic examination of kidneys from the crocks of the Gordon Museum at Guy's Hospital that contained some of the original kidneys described by Bright showed the underlying condition to be related to amyloid, severe arterial vascular disease, and other pathological entities.

Sir Robert Christison's publication in 1839, *On Granular Degeneration of the Kidnies and its Connection with Dropsy, inflammation and other Diseases*, was a slim volume that one might almost be able to place in a deep pocket of a coat, as compared with the large heavy sumptuously bound volume of Bright and the even more oversized volume of Rayer's atlas, containing none of the beautiful lithograph prints of the other two authors. Christison's volume did report on thirty one cases similar to Bright, but several of his cases recovered unlike the universal fatal outcome of all of Bright's cases. Autopsy findings were therefore available in only a little more than half of his cases. The clinical history, pathology and morbid appearance, secondary diseases associated with the renal disease, and a discussion of causes – of which scarlatina was recognized as a factor especially in those that recovered, prognosis and treatment were elaborated upon. Christison's volume and the earlier 1829 report was verified the findings of Bright and expend some of his observations. They outline the causes for the delayed recognition of the condition. The possibility of reversibility of the condition and the demonstration elevated urea in the blood of at least one patient, although in very impure form, was a significant advance.

Jonathan Osborn of Dublin, Ireland

Moving next to Dublin Ireland, Jonathan Osborne's publication in 1837, *On the Nature and Treatment of Dropsical Diseases accompanied by Coagulable Urine and Suppressed Perspiration,* extends the observations of Bright, presenting 36 cases with a review of the literature up to that point, quoting Dr. Barlow of Bath who had also accepted Bright's conclusions. While exposure to cold and alcohol had been considered a factor in the cause of the condition by Bright and Christison, Osborne emphasized suppressed circulation, cool extremities and absence of sweating and took measures primarily to improve this with baths, sweating, blankets, etc. He also confirmed the finding of reduced urea in the urine and elevated urea in some of the patients, confirming the prior studies of Prevost and Dumas, French authors who had previously noted in dogs dying following a bilateral nephrectomy that the urine was depleted of urea but a high value appeared in the blood. This was the first demonstration of the fact that the kidneys did not produce urea, but only excreted it.

Pierre Rayer in Paris, France

On the Continent in France Pierre Rayer was Professor of Medicine at l'hopital de la Charite. He was the teacher of Claude Bernard, Jean Martin Charcot, Charles Brown Sequard and others. He had already produced a treatise on skin diseases, which is translated into English and has been considered the founder of modern Dermatology. He had done descriptive and epidemiological research into glanders, a disease of horses that can be transmitted to humans causing mucus membrane and skin lesions. But it was his three volume publication, first of a comprehensive atlas of pathological engravings of a wide variety of renal conditions in 1839 and to be followed by a two volume detailed description of a carefully considered catalogue and organization of a wide spectrum of clinical and pathological renal diseases, *Traite des Maladies des Reins et des Alterations de la Secretion Urinaire*. He came from the same pathological-clinical school of Richard Bright where attention to autopsy findings were paramount. As in the case of Bright and Christison, microscopic examination of the pathological material was lacking. Not until the early work of Gabriel Valentin (1810-1883) were microscopic sections of renal tissue available. The work of George Johnson, a student of Bright, in 1852, On the *Diseases of the Kidney* and Jean Martin Charcot's *Lectures on Bright's Disease of the Kidneys* (1878) does present and tries to correlated clinical and microscopic pathological material. Rayer recognized the contribution of Bright in the characterizing of this new renal disease and renamed the disease Nephrite Albumineuse. The first volume of the book consists of a Preface, emphasizing the examination of the urine and a careful characterization of the formed elements seen by microscopy with wonderful hand drawings of red blood cell casts, white and red cells, and crystals of urates, phosphates, and even Hippuric acid and Quinine. An extensive catalogue of the bibliography of the studies in renal disease from the Greeks to 1840 appears at the end of the second volume. However it is in the footnotes (footnotes were more in vogue in the early 19th century as can be seen in their use by Gibbons in *The Rise and Fall of the Roman Empire* until their their use was restricted by articles such as *A Garland of Ibids for Van Wyck Brooks*, by Frank Saltonstall Sullivan and modern usage) of the 121 pages of *Nephrite Albumineus* that Rayer expresses his acceptance of Bright's original contribution and demonstrates his knowledge of prior worker's findings and expresses his critique of their work.

After only one and an eight line on page 97 of this chapter, Rayer begins a long footnote of one and one half pages on the general subject naming the condition. IN rather pedantic fashion he dissects the meaning of *nephritis* and rejects the the designation of Bright, *Diseased kidney in Dropsy*, rejects Christison's *Granular degeneration*, rejects *Renal dropsy*, and rejects *albuminorrhea*, a term considered by his French colleague Martin-Solon. Rayer's last sentence in the footnote states,"Finally it has been suggested that the affliction be called Bright's Disease, and I would have been very inclined to adopt that name, which dedicates the discovery of this famous doctor, would it not have seemed preferable to me to give it a significant scientific name."

Summary

From England, Scotland, Ireland and finally to the Continent as represented by France the concept of a clearly defined disease entity to explain dropsy and coaguable urine by reference to kidney disease came to be established in the relatively brief period of thirteen years, between 1827 with the publication of Bright's *Case Reports* to 1840 with encyclopedic two volume *Nephrite* Albumineuse by Pierre Rayer. The various authors discussed here built one upon the other, often quibbling about matters such as the Specific Gravity of blood or urine during the progress of the disease, or the name by which it should be designated. The establishment of this entity was primarily based on clinical and pathological study with of course a newly found devotion to the study of the urine. The development of chemical analysis of urine and blood was in its infancy; Urea was reluctantly recognized in the blood, there were no microscopes to examine urine or pathological section to evaluate sections of the kidney. Treatment was rather uniform based on depletion therapy, where leaches, laxatives, and blood letting were respected forms of therapy. The careful observation of the patients, detailed description of the clinical course, documentation of the medications used, occasionally coming to what we would consider erroneous conclusions as to successful outcomes related to procedures used, such were fairly uniform and common to all the authors. The English-French connection in this nascent period of laying the foundation for the study of renal disease would soon see a shifting of activity to the East, to Germany for clarification of the underlying pathology, as tissue sections using microscopes became available. Friedrich Theodor Frerichs was an experimental pathologist who gained insights into glomerular physiology and Ludwig Traube applied physiological methodology to clinical problems.

Leadership in renal studies would revert back to Guy's Hospital in London, England where Fredrick Malamod would emphasize the roll of hypertension in the evaluation of Bright's Disease. It would also be the Germans who would develop the physiological concepts that would lead the way for the American workers A.N. Richards, Homer Smith.and others to further the concepts of Cushny and develop the chemical and physiological considerations that have made modern concepts of Nephrology possible.

Chapter Two

A Garland of Ibids: The use of Footnotes in the Medical
Writings of Early Nineteenth Century Authors who
Established Bright's Disease as a Clinical Entity

Footnotes were used sparingly by the Ancient writers
and those in the Renaissance, but began to proliferate in
the Enlightenment according to Anthony Grafton.
Medical writers and specifically the forerunners of
Richard Bright and those who followed him and helped
establish renal disease as a clinical entity relating
Dropsy, Coagulable Urine to Granular Kidneys used
footnotes, but not as consistently as might be expected.
Richard Bright himself wrote his 1827 masterpiece, *Case
Reports* in a flowing narrative style, reminiscent or earlier
writers, eschewing footnotes. Robert Christison and
Pierre Rayer, later authors who helped establish the
clinical entity of Bright's Disease, found footnotes to
their liking and used them to present data not felt
appropriate for the text above or as a running counter to
the text to jar the reader's equilibrium and keep him
following a double discourse. This review will focus on
the use of footnotes in the medical writings that

preceded as well as followed Richard Bright's salient observations.

According to Anthony Grafton in *The Footnote, a Curious History*, "in modern American classical scholarship, footnotes often serve to prove the author's membership in a guild rather than to illuminate or support a particular point. Citations are heaped up, without much regard to their origins or compatibility, in order to make the text above them seem to rest on solid pilings." The Talmud with its extensive use of annotations around all four margins of the text, could be considered a forerunner of the use of footnotes. Edward Gibbon's *Delcine and Fall of the Roman Empire* employs footnotes most infamously such as can be seen in Chapter XXI, page 417 of the second volume where three-quarters of a page of footnotes is used to "trace the singular revolutions of those celebrated words, pagans and paganism." Anthony Grafton points out that Gibbon's footnotes were originally placed in the back of the text as endnotes, until Hume complained to Gibbon's publisher that the " notes should occupy a convenient position, at the foot of the page or in the margin." Grafton further comments that modern use of footnotes to examine all sources, is "like the high whine of the dentist's drill, the low rumble of the footnote on the historian's page reassures; the tedium it inflicts, like the pain inflicted by the drill, is not random but directed, part of the cost that the benefits of modern science and technology exact." I remember as a freshman in a college English writing class, the one page spoof by Frank S. Sullivan, *A Garland of IBIDS for Van Wick Brooks* which had appeared in the New Yorker magazine was used as a model as how not to use footnotes. A recent rereading of this short article demonstrates that three-quarters of the page is occupied by footnotes that respond to and argue among themselves with the main section of the report.

Footnotes occasionally make their appearance in current textbooks of medicine or in journal articles. Endnotes to document the citation of pertinent listing of references are of course commonplace. In examining the very first page of Pierre Rayer's chapter *Nephrite Albumineuse* in the second volume of *Traite* des *Maladies des Reins*, one is initially reminded of Sullivan spoof. Immediately after the title, *Nephrite Albumineuse*, before the text has had a chance to proclaim itself, there is a full two pages of footnotes! Actually this gigantic footnote is very much to the point in that it discusses in detail the proper name that should be applied to the relatively new clinical syndrome described by Richard Bright only thirteen years earlier in 1827; ie. Bright's publication of *Reports of Medical Cases selected with a view of illustrating The Symptoms and Cure of Diseases by reference to Morbid Anatomy.* Rayer's footnote was not unique to medical reports in the early nineteenth century. It will be shown that the followers of Bright in developing this new concept of a disease linking dropsy, coagulable urine and granular kidneys, Robert Christison, Jonathan Osborne, and Pierre Rayer used footnotes extensively. They helped form a running dialogue to their often dry repetitive text. It was in the footnotes that editorial comments from past authors are displayed, commented upon negatively or praised, where important new data is to be found, and in truth where the real substance of the topic is pitted against the accompanying rumbling text.

Footnotes as found in Richard Bright's 1827 Reports of Medical Cases

Remarkably enough the document that established the entity of Bright's disease, *Reports of Medical* Cases in 1827 contains no footnotes in comparison with the supporting reports and volumes that followed Bright. Perhaps a truly original work that sets out an entirely new concept requires less of the scholarly annotation of sources that footnotes imply. More likely Bright preferred the uninterrupted narrative style of the earlier authors of the Ancients and Renaissance. In the introduction to the Case Reports, Bright does give credit in the text itself, not in a footnote to Dr. Blackall (John Blackall-1771-1860 *Observations on the Nature and Cure of Dropsies and Particularly on the Presence of the Coagulable Part of the Blood in Dropsical Urine* 1813), "The observations which I have made respecting the condition of the urine in dropsy, are in a great degree in accordance with what has been laid down by Dr. Blackall in his most valuable treatise." Richard Bright could have given credit to William Charles Wells' 1812 report in *Transactions of a Society for the Improvement of Medical and Chirurgical Knowledge, On the presence of the red Matter and Serum of Blood in the Urine of Dropsy, which has not originated from Scarlet Fever.* Very few footnotes are used in this publication as well, and Wells, like Bright chooses to give credit in the text itself to a still earlier author Cruikshank in Rollo's *Treatise on Diabetes (1798)*, where there is described "the urine in dropsy often contains serum." Bright does incorporate into his text three letters from John Bostock documenting chemical analysis of urine and blood from Bright's patients. Such information would have been found in the voluminous footnotes of Christison and Rayer, who were to follow and confirm the original work of Bright. Richard Bright would give credit in the body of his report to Thomas Hodgkin and James Alderson who had referred several cases for study, but declined the use of footnotes for such purposes. Such acknowledgements and information would find their way into footnotes in the writings of many of the authors that would follow Bright. We leave Richard Bright's monumental and incisive work without a footnote to comment upon. If footnotes really counted, Bright would probably not be recognized today.

Footnotes as used by Sir Robert Christison in Publications of 1829 and 1939

Sir Robert Christison, physician at the Royal Infirmary in Edinburgh, was the first to confirm and champion the observations of Richard Bright in two publication of 1829 and 1839, that would provide a plethora of *garland of ibids* for study! The earlier publication *Observation on the Variety of Dropsy which Depends on Kidney Disease,* in 1829 two years after Bright's original observation in *Case Reports,* points out in the body of the text that, "no other physician (other than himself) has publicly noticed his discovery or endeavored to confirm or extend his statement that dropsy appears to originate in organic derangement of the kidney and is one of the frequent varieties of this disease." This 1829 report consists of detailed descriptions of seven cases very similar to the reports of Bright. In footnotes to Case 1, Robert Irving, is detailed chemical analysis of the urine that had not previously been documented in a clinical setting. Berzelius in 1812 had isolated and quantitated crystals of urea in urine, as had William Prout, one of the Animal Chemist working with Richard Bright. From this Case 1 the urine is analyzed on two separate occasions, and what is most striking, values from control subjects, or as Christian calls them, "healthy urine" are also recorded. The items studied in the urine consisted of Specific Gravity, Volume of Urine, Urea /animal Acetate, Solids, Alkaline Murates, Sulfate/Phosphate, Earthy Phosphates, Vesical mucous, and Albumin. While the methodology of how these items were determined and the reliability of the methods are vague, the footnotes provide a beginning for clinical urinalysis that takes account of more chemical determinations than is the custom for a urinalysis today. In a separate footnote is the effect of phlebotomy on these parameters of "urinalysis", as well as a similar chemical reports in another footnote on a second case. While not included in the footnotes but rather in the body of the report is the first description of a an isolation and characterization of crystals of urea from urine, up until then not recognized in normal urine nor convincingly demonstrated in renal failure.

The use of footnotes in Robert Christison's *On Granular Degereration of the Kidnies and its Connection with Dropsy, Inflammations and other Diseases* of 1839, a book of 144 pages with a preface, would become more florid with long dialogues on the observations of others and strongly held opinions of the author. *Granular Degeneration of the Kidnies* (Christison's spelling of kidneys) summaries an additional 31 cases fulfilling the criteria of Bright with the findings of dropsy, coagulable urine found in the presence of renal pathology, which Christison prefers to label granular degeneration, from the gross appearance of the diseased kidneys. His indebtedness to Richard Bright is acknowledged. Footnotes are added to the section on the history of the development of the condition over the past 12 years since Bright's original publication. These are laid out in a straight forward fashion, citing the author's name and the reference ie: J. Osborne, *On the Nature and Treatment of Dropsical Diseases*, 1834, Pierre Rayer, *Nephrite Albumineuse 1837,* etc, etc without elaboration or comment, much as footnotes would be used to cite pertinent references in a current medical text. In the next section however, Christison warms up to his task of using footnotes as a counter and independent voice in the narrative. In a long footnote of one third of a page is a discussion of the opinions of Rayer, M. Solon (a French colleague of Rayer), Gregory (a Scotch colleague of Christian), etc on the varieties of pathology noted in the kidneys: congestive, granular, atrophic indurated, tuberculosis, etc. Then there is reported in a footnote a medical legal case- "a woman of stout muscular form of tolerable sound health and somewhat given to intoxication who died not long after a squabble with her husband. Marks of contusion were on the body and base of the brain, but also very far advance granular degeration in the kidneys." The cause of death remained in some doubt, trauma or granular degeneration of the kidney?

A short footnote appears concerning the color of the urine, "Care must be taken as Mr. Rees (one of the physician chemists working with Bright) has suggested not to mistake for a feature of the disease, the colours imparted to the urine by many articles of vegetables." With regard to a discussion of Specific Gravity in various stages of the disease, Christison comments in a footnote of seventeen lines, "Far to little attention has been paid by most authors to the density of the urine. The French writers in particular, seemed to have greatly neglected it, (Rayer's discussion of SpG in and out of footnotes however is extensive) and to have erroneous notions of its condition and import. M. Solon appears to hold that the density is always greatly reduced, where it is certainly far from being the fact, and no French author seems to have correct ideas of the relation which the density bears to the progress of the disease, etc." Christison usually very urbane, doesn't usually exhibit such Scottish petulance, but he and other observers paid a considerable attention to SpG, perhaps because it was one of the few easily performed quantitative analysis available.

The longest footnote, three pages, appears on pages 18-21, in response to the query as to whether liver disease without accompanying renal disease can be responsible for coagulable urine, "It would tend greatly to perplex the reader if I entered in the text a full examination of the various facts and statements which have lately been put forward by authors in contradiction to the general principals laid down above. (ie: that fixed chronic coagulable urine implies granular kidneys) But it may be right to admit more particularly the question in a note." This is probably the best excuse to employ a "note" ie: footnote, rather than entangle the narrative with ancillary material. Christison then goes on in detail in this footnote to discuss the unlikely presence of coagulable urine without renal disease being present: Citing J. Osborne, "healthy urine doesn't contain coaguable urine, but it may occur occasionally." Rayer is cited in studies of "400 healthy or recovering patients surveyed at random and only in three was there coagulable urine in the absence of granular kidneys. Similarly M. Solon evaluated 500-600 in health, finding only one with coaguable urine, etc"

On page 21, in describing the best way of demonstrating coagulable urine (classically described by Bright as holding a spoon over a candle) in a long footnote Christison describes a more elegant technique for semi quantitative analysis." The best way of operating (ie: testing for albumin) is with a tube about a third of an inch in diameter, a spoon which many use, is a clumsy substitute, which will not show the nicer degree of coagulably." (one of the few occasions Christison has a negative comment on his idol Bright). Continuing in the footnote and attempting a graded semiquantitative analysis: "Common nomenclature for degree of coagulability 1)Gelation by heat, 2)Very strongly coagulable, loaded with flakes, 3) Strongly coagulable precipitate in 24 hours occupying half volume of fluid, 4) Moderately coagulable – occupying ¼ of the fluid, 5) Slight coagulable 1/8 of volume. 6) Hazy by heat – where urine becomes cloudy with no flakes." And finally there is a most astute observation universally observed today, all in the footnote, "In appreciating the last degree of impregnation, it is convenient to heat only the upper half of the fluid in the tube."

Footnotes commonly may be used to cite pertinent references. In the case of the authors under consideration, those who established and confirmed the clinical entity of Bright's Disease, footnotes were more commonly used to provided valuable and original information. Christison's information on the composition of urine in healthy and diseased states is of this variety. Alternatively they may be used to take to task their colleagues, encouraging them to accept the author's opinions or cajole them in accepting his view point. This later use of footnotes is to be found in Christison's ¾ page of footnotes on page 25 of *Granular Degeneration*. Considering the question of " the proportion of albumin in the urine necessarily increasing as the disease advances, the very opposite is the general rule." Christison then footnotes the following remarks. "Among others, M. Solon seems to have fallen into this mistake…that the secretion of albumin is vicarious with the secretion of urea" (vicarious meaning unrelated). Christison continuing in the footnote then quotes his own data to show that in advanced disease the urine is dilute, low SpG, low urea and small amount of albumin, emphasizing his   position that "albumin abounds most in the early stages and decreases in the advanced stage." He then goes on in his characteristic fashion of mixing clinical observation with chemical analysis and cajoling his colleagues to reconsider their findings in the light of his observations,   all in this footnote, "I have been so careful in my observation upon the accuracy of ocular inspection of the urine along with repeated chemical analysis…..that I feel almost inclined to express the hope that those eminent authors (that disagree with him) will repeat their experiments on the relative coagulability of the urine in different stages of the disease. Should their original statements be then verified,   there is need to consider several varieties of the disease and there would be the need to establish the exact relationship subsisting between coagulability and the several degrees and variety." Christison sticks by the reliability of his observation, encourages his colleagues, "eminent authors", to repeat their observations feeling they will see the error of their ways and agree with him, but if not, the way out is to recognized they are not discussing the same disease, that there may exist, "the several varieties of the disease." In any event it will be important to "establish the exact relationship subsisting between coagulability and the several degrees and variety" (of diseases)

This problem that Bright's disease might represent several varieties of an underlying disease processes and that dogmatic statements about the characteristics of the condition may vary with the underlying process was considered a possibility early on. Having only gross pathological and the primitive chemical studies of the urine and blood, holding that Bright's disease was a monolithic entity was certain to bring confusion. Pathological specimens of Bright's kidneys stored in the Gordon Pathological Museum at Guys Hospital were studied by A. Arnold Osman by microscopic sections in the 20th century and proved to be a mixture of amyloid, vascular disease, etc. Christison's emphasis on detailed observation, establishment of standards and admitting to the possibilities of Bright's disease being a mixed bag of clinical and pathological entities explaining why "eminent authors" could come to different conclusions, all is recorded in the ¾ page of footnote on page 25 of *Granular Degeneration*.

As an introduction to his next large detailed footnote of 60 lines or about four fifth of page 32, is the statement in the text that "the early stages of the disease is characterized by the low density of its serum, defective proportion of albumin, by the frequent presence of urea, by frequent increase in fibrin and by the proportion of the haematosin (hemoglobin) being unaffected." It is here that Christison seems to feel obliged to let the reader in on the exact method of analysis of the items he has mentioned, fibrin, haematosin, serum, and albumin. He does this in a detailed and exacting footnote and justifiying the reason for putting it in the form of a footnote right from the start. "In order not to interrupt the train of statement given above (that is in the text itself), I shall here subjoin the method of analysis." With this statement Christison tips his hand as to why he employs footnotes, ie: in "order not to interrupt the train of statements given above", since as will be seen, if this methodological diversion would be a part of the text, he would likely lose many of his readers right then and there because of its length and complexity. Christison continues, "On some occasions the blood was collected in a bottle containing a few fragments of lead, and the bottle after being filled to the lip, secured with a grooved stopper, and agitated for 10 minutes. It was then weighed to ascertain the quantity of blood made use of. The fibrin, which was all collected around the lead, was then separated, well squeezed, slightly washed, squeezed again, and weighted moist. It was next well soaked in repeated portions of water to remove the serum, which may well be supposed to constitute its impregnating fluid and lastly dried in the vapour bath till it ceased to lose weight. This gave the amount of dry fibrin" After all that squeezing, drying, washing and weighing Christison has a value for the fibrin in the sample. He goes on in similar fashion, with the fibrin being removed to employ similar tedious procedures to quantitatively separate and weigh the serum, albumin and finally the hematosin. The laborious attention to details is certainly appreciated even if the errors of the method are not addressed. This very method for estimating these items was taken over almost verbatim by Rayer, also in an extended footnote in his chapter *Nephrite Albumineurs* in *Traite des Maladies des Reins*, as will be indicated later.

On page 34 of *Granular Degeneration* Christison takes on the effect of blood letting on the composition of the blood in a footnote of 5/8 of a page. Data from two patients and a healthy control are presented. The normal Hematosin value (roughly related to Hgb) falls from a control value of 12.07gm to 5.74 and 5.77 gms respectively after vigorous use of phlebotomy, as was commonly employed at that time. His conclusions are that Hematosin levels are "greatly reduced by blood letting, slowly regenerated and the solids in the blood are increased." A case of a middle age female with hypertrophy of the heart and palpations followed by pneumonia, both considered to display "inflammation" and require blood letting is illustrative of the changes in Fibrin, Solids, Urates, and the dramatic changes in Hematosin noted above, all in this extended footnote, documenting the changes in the blood, but failing to question the salutary effects of the procedure.

In a relatively brief footnote on Dropsy of 10 lines on page 38 of *Granular Degeneration*, Christison comments that, "some pathologists, especially in France, incorrectly consider anasarca as an essential characteristic of the disease." Christison quotes Bright to substantiate this opinion in this same footnote, "the contrary is shown by the experience of Dr. Bright as well as by the frequent observation at the Edinburgh Infirmary. The disease, says Dr. Bright may exist in all its force and be fatal without the effusion of a single drop of fluid in the cellular membranes at any period of its course (citing Bright), *Guy's Hospital Report*, 1838, vol ii." Rayer, being referred to as "some pathologists, especially in France", in a footnote in his *Traite des Reins*, in describing the importance of anasarca to the diagnosis of the condition states, "Dr. Christison was wrong, it seems to me, to classify the anasarca among *secondary ailments*; in the acute state, dropsy is one of the most constant

phenomena and the most characteristic of the disease."
The interplay of Christison and Rayer discussing this
nascent diagnosis of renal disease will have many
opportunities to jockey back and forth their views,
agreeing with each other or vigorously countering each
others opinion on many aspects of this new clinical
entity. Rayer will have his turn to develop his views on
the significance of anasarca as well as a variety of other
controversial subjects, as well as to argue with and at
times to praise the English doctors about their
understanding of a clinical entity that had been
introduced by Richard Bright only about threteen years
earlier.

Footnotes have been demonstrated to be used by Dr.
Christison in his 1839 volume *Granular Degeneration* to
provide valuable early chemical data from analysis of
blood and urine, chastise his colleagues and "eminent
authors" for opinions not supported by himself, but
willing to reverse these staunchly held opinions, if the
data proves otherwise. Christison's footnotes are a
veritable early textbook of nephrology in themselves.

Footnotes as found in Publications of James Craufurd Gregory, 1831 and 1832

James Craufurd Gregory was a colleague of Robert
Christison at the Royal Infirmary of Edinburgh. He
unfortunately died at the age of 32 of typhus. (or
possibly typhoid since the two diseases were not clearly
differentiated at that time in England) They shared
cases and referred to each other in their publications.
They both referred to the literature on Dropsy and
Albuminuria primarily through Bright's publication.
They both quoted the work of Wells, Blackall and
Cruickshank. And yet their respective handling of
footnotes were worlds apart. It was as if Gregory had
been writing in the late twentieth century. Footnotes,

yes, but they are employed in a controlled fashion, not to dazzle the reader with new or controversial information or to engage in long polemics as has been seen with Christison and will be seen in the writings of John Osborne and Pierre Rayer. The use of footnotes with James Craufurd Gregory are straight forward citing of references to the literature, without embellishment or comment. Gregory's use of footnotes can be seen by his review of the literature prior to Bright's publication of 1827. Gregory cites three authors, 1) Van Helmont, "who distinctly lays down the kidneys as the seat of the disease in dropsy" and lists as a footnote, *Ortus Medicinae, Cap. Ignotus Hydrops,* 2) Morgagni, "who described anasarca followed by diarrhoea, in which no organ was found diseased except the kidney," citing in a footnote *De Sed. Et Caus. Morg., Epist. Xl11, Art. 11.* and finally at the bottom of this page 3) Charles William Wells, "has given (described) only three cases of persons who had died dropsical with coagulable urine, whose bodies were examined after death; and in all three the kidneys were found diseased.", citing the appropriate referernce in a footnote. Continuing in the text, Gregory states, "Yet he (Wells) draws no inference from these facts, and thinks it necessary to state, that he does not conclude from the appearances that the kidneys are always diseased, when the urine in dropsy contains much serum, and that the morbid appearances in the kidneys might be altogether unconnected with the morbid secretion." (Wells did not feel he had enough evidence to positively implicate dropsy and coagulable urine with kidney abnormalities since several of the kidneys examined were relatively normal and few autopsy specimens were examined.) The footnote referring to Wells is neatly recorded at the bottom of the page beneath the other two authors, and cited as *Transactions of a Society for the Improvement of Medical and Chirurgical Knowledge, Vo. 111, 1812, Read 1811.* The title of the article, <u>On the presence of the red</u>

Matter and Serum of Blood in the Urine of Dropsy, which has not originated from the Scarlet Fever, is not referred to in the footnote, but is quoted in the body of the text. These three footnotes designated with typographical symbols, rather than numerical designations are without additional comment or discussion, unlike some other authors of the day.

Footnotes as Found in the Publication of Authors Preceding Richard Bright

1. William Charles Wells 1812

William Charles Wells was an American born in South Carolina whose sympathies with British during our Revolutionary War drove him to leave America and to continue to practice medicine in England, working at St Thomas Hospital in London, He almost made the correlation that would be the prize of Richard Bright. Gregory attributes his failure to make the correlation between dropsy, coaguable urine and kidney disease to, stating in the text, "these authors (Van Helmont, Morgagni, and Wells) apparently led away by the preconceived notion of dropsy being in most cases at least, a general disease of the system without local affection (disease), and have neglected to draw the very obvious conclusion to which their own cases would naturally lead."

Wells use of footnotes in his paper *On the presence of the red Matter and Serum of Blood in the Urine of Dropsy* is sparse and without acknowledgment to any past authors. The only exceptions are three rather lengthy footnotes or asides, the first on p. 217 of one third of the page, indicating that more frequently urine containing serum (albumin). is in men rather than in woman, which he attributes to the finding being "accidental ."

This was probably not an accidental finding but correctly points out the predominance of male to females with acute glomerulonephritis. The second footnote of more than a page in length describes the findings at autopsy of an "elderly man labouring some time under a disease in his chest, and dropsy of the skin (edema) whose urine had contained considerable quantity of serum. The kidnies (Wells spelling as well as Christison) were larger and softer than if in a healthy state,.. and about fifteen pints of fluid in the abdomen .. which when exposed to heat, the coagulum formed was very great." Wells was unwilling to relate the appearance of the kidnies to the presence of dropsy. The third and last rather brief footnote on p. 232 discusses the advisability of the use of cantharides, or dried Spanish fly, a powerful blistering agent and possible diuretic, in patients with dropsy. For the most part however, Well's long rambling paper follows the discursive narrative form in the style of Richard Bright.

2. John Blackall 1813

As mentioned in the introduction, John Blackall's *Observations on the Nature and Cure of Dropsies, and Particularly on the Presence of the Coagulable Part of the Blood in Dropsical Urine first published in 1813*, is the only historical   reference Richard Bright credits in his 1827 *Case Reports.*   Blackall's *Observations* is a rambling 274 pages on the finding, as stated in the Introduction, "in a considerable number of dropsical cases in which the urine coagulates like diluted serum of the blood." Blackall was a physician to the Devon and Exeter Hospital and to the lunatic asylum near Exeter. He initiates his discussion with an extensive historical account that Richard Bright found reason to ignore. The footnotes to this historical introduction are succinctly listed, often with an incompleteness that would leave the modern reader in ignorance as to how to locate such references. He lists in footnotes, as just a representative sampling: 1. Latham on Diabetes, p. 139, 2. Darwin's Zoonamia vol, 1st volume p316; on quoting the findings of the French chemists-physicians Vauqulin and Forcroy's finding of gelatinous matter and albumin in human urine, the reference is given as 3. *Annales de Chimie: tom 31 and 33*. Blackall continues in the text giving credit to "Mr. Cruichshank in his appendix to Dr. Roll's excellent work on Diabetes, "noting the serous urine more precisely than any other author has done," designating as a footnote, 4. see Appendix to Rollo on Diabetes, p.447 and 448. All of these references show an exhaustive search of the literature as well as many additional citations including Boerhaave's Aphorisms and Withering's account of the Foxglove. Such listings could be considered as the use of footnotes, according to Anthony Grafton "to prove the author's membership in a guild rather then to illuminate or support a particular point. Citations are heaped up, without much regard to their origins or compatibility in order to make the text above seem to rest on solid pilings." The absence of date of publication of these references and other identifying information would probably not pass muster of a modern day editor however.

The most extended footnote appears in the discussion on the likelihood that dropsical accumulations may supply the albumin appearing in the urine in many cases. Blackall states in the body of the text that the "kidney from the comparative simplicity of their secretions are probably the gland most suited to such an office. They seem to be possessed of a sort of selective power capable of separating from the blood whatever is hurtful of it. The urine is perpetually impregnated both in smell and colour with foreign material." While this physiological speculation seems unusual, the concept that the kidney could contribute albumin to the urine as part of a pathological process by itself seems foreign to Blackall's thinking. But then he argues against this theory pointing out that coaguable urine may appear when there is the total absence of dropsy. To illustrate this fact Blackall tells the tale of a patient with "imaginary syphilis"in a long footnote of three quarters of a page in length. This footnote explains that by "imaginary syphilis" he refers to a patient who believed he had this disease and "earnestly desired to take mercury" although Blackall thought he had already taken enough since apparently the patient had already shown signs of coagulable urine and had other symptoms of excess mercury. In addition to his hypochondriasis over his belief that he required even more mercury, he had developed "irritation of the urinary organs, vomiting in the middle of the night of a black bile and undigested food, frothy stools and excessive emaciation and despondency." Continuing in this voluminous footnote, Blackall explains that on examination after death no cause was found for the coagulable urine, the "whole disease was caused by a cicatrized ulcer near the cardia of the stomach the size of a shilling. Every thing else was sound and in order." This long case history in this footnote supported the proposition therefore that dropsy need not be the only factor contributing to coagulable urine. Blackall seems to have missed the opportunity to speculate on the possibility of mercury was contributing to coagulable urine, since by the statement "every thing else was sound and in order," he overlooked the kidney as a source of proteinuria. Whether mercury was commonly a factor in coaguable urine would be considered by Bright, Rayer, and others. Except for this protracted case history in the form of a footnote, Blackall's early footnotes were succinct, crisp, to the point, and cognizant of prior authors, even if details of the references were often lacking.

Footnotes as found in the Publication of Jonathan Osborne from 1834

Jonathan Osborne (1775-1864), recognized as Ireland's first Nephrologist, published a slim volume entitled "On the Nature and Treatment of Dropsical Diseases." He was very much impressed by the finding of "suppressed perspiration" as a major factor in the development of dropsy and vigorously promulgated measures to counteract it, such as hot and steam baths, including the immersion of an extremity in a vapour bath. He very much accepted the findings of Richard Bright on the relationship of dropsy, albuminuria and underlying kidney disease and the first 42 pages of his text details the history of the disease, citing Wells, Blackall, Bright, Christison and even the French workers, Prevost and Dumas who had removed the kidneys from an animal and found the blood urea to progressively rise, demonstrating conclusively and for the first time that the kidney did not make urea but excreted it. All these sources are detailed in the body of the text without a single footnote! Beginning on page 43 however there commences a series of footnotes, while not rivaling those used by Christison or Rayer (to be review shortly), are used not only to cite prior references but to engage in asides and present material with which the author perhaps didn't want to clutter up the body of the text.

On page 43 of Osborne's text there are two brief footnotes with regard to treatment. The first with regard to the timing of warm baths, "I have seen some practitioners prefer the employment of warm baths in the AM .... the greater tendency to perspire in an individual at night and during sleep renders the hour of going to bed more expeditious." The second brief footnote on this same page refers to treatment recommending the "peculiar properties of treacle (a sugar and molasses remedy) better known to common

people than among the facility to promote sweating."
On page 48 is a footnote of one half a page on iodine
usage in dropsy. Further on is an interesting brief
footnote on the use of leeches into the rectum in dropsy,
"to unload the vessels of the venaportae." Osborne
continues in this footnote, "In the Dublin Medical
Journal I have described a convenient mode of
introducing leeches into the rectum by securing them
with silk threads attached to the groves of an instrument
prepared for the purpose." The longest of Osborne's
footnotes, two and one half pages, is in the section
related to vascular and cardiac causes of dropsy,
describing the pulse primarily in aortic valvular disease.
The etiology of such valvular disease are considered to
include "direct pressure from without, such as the
shoemaker resting the last on the sternum of his left side
or the tailor in this country constantly stooping forward
at their work, both are peculiarly prone to diseases of the
aortic valve!"

Pierre Rayer Footnotes in his Traite des Maladies des Reins et des Alterations de la Secretion Urinaire

Pierre Rayer (1793-1867) considered the founder of
French Nephrology, published between 1839 and 1841 a
two volume *Traite des Maladies des Reins* of over *2100
pages* and a large Atlas of renal pathology. The end of
the second volume of *Traite* contains over 100 hundred
pages on a detailed history of renal disease from
antiquity to the nineteenth century, the dawn of the
recognition of renal disease by Bright and others. The
first volume of the *Traite* consists of a *Preface* and a
Prolegomena, the latter an antiquated designation for an
introduction and critical evaluation of methods in
examining the urine, measurement of urea, etc. Tissue
sections of renal pathology were yet to be developed,
physiological concepts of renal function were to be

developed later in the century, and the microscope even for examination of urine was just beginning to be employed by Rayer as can be seen in his plates describing casts and formed elements, as well as Quinine crystals which he was the first to describe. Gabriel Richet has detailed Rayer's contribution to the emerging field of renal disease, emphasizing his innovative method of clinical investigation. Rayer contributed relatively little original knowledge to the budding field of renal disease, in comparison to Bright and Christison, but he masterfully examined the field critically, and had a profound knowledge of all the investigators in the field, commenting upon them sometimes favorably and at others time with questioning disdain. The text demonstrates Rayer's extensive clinical experience with renal disease although his therapeutic maneuvers represent monotonous and commonly used remedies shared by the physicians of the times, such as the use of bizarre and potent laxative, leeches, bleeding, etc.

Rayer's *Traite* has even today not been translated into English nor has Bright's *Case Reports* been translated into French. An examination of the footnotes of Rayer's second volume of the *Traite,* considering his long chapter on *Nephrite Albumineus,* will demonstrate his robust use of footnotes to amplify and critically examine the work of his predecessors, and as with Christison to present new data of utmost interest and importance. Rayer's footnotes are used not so much to cite and document pertinent references, since the field was relatively new and only a limited number of investigators are to be contended with, but rather to serve as a running commentary to the main body of the text, that would allow an editorial voice that could comment independently on the text.

As mentioned in the Introduction of this paper, Rayer's use of Footnotes caught my attention after only reading the title of the chapter, Nephrite Albumineuse. This footnote could be a turn off for a casual reader, a gigantic aside, that could divert attention from the text itself, even before a single sentence is read. To the contrary, this footnote of two entire pages is very much to the point and the substance of the footnote could be translated into Shakespearian English as, "What's in a name?"

What should we call this new disease, described by Richard Bright, characterized by dropsy, coagulable urine, and abnormalties of kidneys at autopsy? Rayer defends his appellation, Albuminous nephritis. He points out that using a term like nephritis, implying inflammation, is appropriate. He emphasized the need to recognize the acute form of the disease (Bright had primarily described the chronic form of the disease, presenting autopsy confirmation in all but three of his cases). Christison had already pointed out the importance of acute potentially reversible forms of the condition. Rayer discusses other designation for the disease, *Diseased Kidney in Dropsy*, Bright 1827, *Granular Degeneration of the Kidnies*, Christison, *The diseased states of the kidney connected during life with albuminous urine*, favored by Gregory. Rayer indicates in this mamouth footnote that he has found them all wanting. "The name *albuminorrhea*, proposed by Martin-Solon (a French colleague) is even more defective." And finally Rayer both magnanimously and with scientific concern considers, "It has been suggested that the affliction be called *Bright's disease*, and I would have been very inclined to adopt that name, which dedicates the discovery of this famous doctor, would it not have seemed preferable to me to give it a significant scientific name."

The majority of Rayer's footnotes appear in the first 62 pages of the discussion of *Nephrite Albumineuse* and vary in length from two pages, as seen above to the merest quoting of a single reference line. The subject matter and variety of the footnotes vary and the following are representative samples of Rayer's unique use of footnotes to editorialized and complement his text.

Concerning the *Anatomical characteristics,* Rayer in a rather ponderous dogmatic way describes *six categories or forms,* in a footnote," Dr. Bright described three of them which seem to me to correspond to our third, fourth and sixth forms, and he indicated another. Dr. Martin-Solon has adopted my divisions, however he joined in a single form the fourth and fifth forms. Dr. Christison admitted seventh forms, but here is one which appears to me entirely foreign to the disease."

In the text Rayer refers to Bright's beautiful colored plates describing the *granulated texture of the kidneys,* "Bright had described a large heavier kidney, the exterior surface, most often a pale yellow, scattered and sometimes covered with small spots of *Milk white"* Here Rayer inserts a footnote to object to the *English doctor's* choice of words for the color of the kidney, "The designation of *yellowish granular matter* used by most English doctors does not give an exact idea for most of the ordinary granulations."

Rayer in making the point that Nephrite Albumineuse, or Bright's Disease as he is willing to call it, is usually a painless affair (unlike calculus or infection in the bladder) In a footnote, Rayer pounces on Sir Robert Christison's statement that "almost all the patients experience pain while urinating, frequent desire to urinate but can only do so with difficulty" Continuing in the same footnote, Rayer sites the appropriate reference to Christison, *On granular degeneration of the kidnies, London 1839.- Edinb.med. and surg. journ. vol XXXVll.* Rayer then continues in this same footnote

"*That opinion, which I do not believe to be exact, was perhaps suggested to him by a small number of dropsy cases with coagulable urine (Gregory, Obs.LXl) where this phenomenon has been observed, and by some other cases of urinary tract disease, distinctly different from albuminous nephritis, and which, wrongly, have been considered as belonging to that disease.*" The footnote is a clear barb at Christison whom he accuses of not recognizing that pain and frequence is a relatively infrequent presenting symptom and that Christison may have mistakingly diagnosed other kidney conditions with that set of symptoms.

Christison while describing beautifully the progression of symptoms in acute and chronic renal failure with many of its complications, does stress these local symptoms, perhaps to a degree that Rayer is not altogether unfair in his criticism. Christison lists, "local pain and other local uneasiness" as the initial symptoms of *Granular Disorganization of Kidnies*. In the body of the Text, Christison describes the acute initial symptoms, "after exposure to cold or wet, the urine becomes scant, highly albuminous and bloody, there also is for the most part frequent desire to pass urine, at time difficulty or positive pain in discharging it, not uncommonly dull, more rarely acute pain in the loins, aggravated by pressure and sometimes shooting downwards to the inside of the thighs or external parts of generation- and more usually pain across the pit of the stomach and in the flanks either felt only on pressure or increased by it, but constantly present more or less." This emphasis on local symptoms is not entirely supported by a review of the thirty one cases presented. Frequency, pain in the loins and difficulty with micturation were recorded as a sole finding or sometime in combination in eleven of these case reports, but only one had lower pelvic pain that warranted sounding the bladder for a stone, which was not found. Autopsies were obtained in only four of these eleven with symptoms. Obs LXI of Dr. James

Gregory, William Graham,did have "scanty, bloody, painful micturition" and Gregory was "disposed to place some reliance in this disease" on the symptom of "pain referred to the lumbar region" Gregory reports that almost half of his forty-six cases had such symptoms, but autopsies were infrequent and many recovered without confirmed diagnosis.

After taking to task Christison on one or two other points, Rayer gives him credit for pointing out that urea may be found elevated in the blood in some cases of the disease. While urea could be measured in the urine, it was unusual in healthy individuals and even in renal failure to be able to measure any urea in the blood. Indeed it was Christison who was the first to publish, and in a footnote at that, previously quoted, the finding of elevated urea in the blood of several of his patients. It is to this point that Rayer gives credit to Dr. Christison stating in a footnote, "Indeed, Dr. Christison reports an observation which proves that urea can exist very early on in the blood of individuals suffering from that disease."

Just before the next footnote, but unfortunately not in a footnote, is the very astute and I believe original observation on the bubbles that appear in nephrotic urine, "When one examines a test tube filled with albuminous urine, one almost always sees, on the surface and against the sides, a certain number of bubbles; and if one adds air to the urine using a tube or a blow pipe, large bubbles form instantly that look like those that children make with soap."

To proceed with this next footnote almost a page in length, but not as clear or succinct as the above observation, Rayer describes the various effects of adding Nitric acid and/or heat to albuminous urine. "After having precipitated with nitric acid, the albumin in the urine, an excess of acid is added, the albuminous flakes almost always pucker, and the precipitate appears less abundant than previously...if one adds a large excess of concentrated nitric acid, the precipitate formed by a few drops of this same acid, dissolves completely or almost completely. If one adds a certain quantity of water to the mixture, the urine becomes cloudy again and the flakes of albumin reappear. But when is has been coagulated by heat, the albumin contained in these urines never become completely transparent through the excess of nitric acid." Further studies on the color of the precipitated albumin are described.

There then follows in this same footnote a simple experiment to determine whether the albumin in the urine is similar to egg albumin. "If with the urine (presumably normal urine) one mixes the white of an egg dissolved in water and filtered", the same effects with Nitric acid and heat described with albuminous urine occur. The minor difference between the reaction of albuminous urine and when egg albumin is added to normal urine are listed, but there is enough similarity in reaction to convince the reader that the material that precipitates in *Nephrite albumineurs* is really albumin. Bright had also described in detail the flocculation of urine "held in a spoon over a candle" but the chemical manipulations described in this footnote of Rayer are more elegant.

As if to apologize to Dr. Christison for his critical remarks earlier cited, Rayer in a footnote of almost a page in length, quoting him almost verbatim, gives him utmost credit for the studies Christison had previously detailed in his own footnote on the composition of the blood in renal disease concerning the measurement of fibrin albumin and serum and hemotosin (heme) which was detailed earlier in the section on Robert Christison. Rayer skips over that initial delightful explaination as to why Christison placed these remarks in the form of a footnote, "in order not to interrupt the train of the statement given above." Rayer may placed his quotation of Christison in a footnote for just such reason however. "Dr. Christison who especially devoted himself to the study of the relative proportions of the organic elements of the blood of dropsy patients whose urine is coagulable, uses the following procedure, as the one most helpful in arriving at this determination. The blood is collected, *spurting from the vein*, in a bottle with a *ground glass stopper*. It is weighed in order to assure the quantity of blood with which one is working. Then the bottle is shaken; the fibrin which has accumulated around the fragments of lead is separated out, and after having been compressed, washed and compressed a second time it is weighed while still moist." (the words in italics represent the difference in Rayer's translation of Christian to his French.) Rayer continues in this footnote quoting further the procedure of Christison on the chemical determinants of the blood, almost exactly.

On the next page there appears a half page footnote on the subject of the low serum albumin almost universally reported in these patients with dropsy and heavy proteinuria. " This diminution of the proportion of albumin was first noticed by Drs. Bostock, Christison, and Gregory." Rayer continues in this same footnote quoting the observations of these authors as well as Bright, and Babington (the English and Scottish observers) on the reduced Specific Gravity of the of serum in renal disease.

Finally there are the footnotes on page 131 and 132 on the controversy over whether mercury can be a contributing factor to albuminuria and renal disease. In his characteristic thorough and historical approach to the subject and with a few observations his own, Rayer tackles the subject, in footnotes, of course. The historical aspect of this problem is addressed in a footnote referring to the observations of Wells, who Rayer quotes as concluding that, "mercury administed in a high dose can cause the excretion of serum (albumin) in the urine. In the substance of the text, Rayer states, "Mercurial preparation have been accused of producing dropsy with coagulable urine; but the cases in which this fact was observed are too few in number to allow one to admit that mercury, unless administered in a very high dosage, and even then in exceptional cases, be a cause of the affection of the kidneys. For many years I have used a plethora of mercurial preparations in treating skin diseases (Rayer had published a well known text and atlas on Skin Diseases) and liver disorders, without ever having noticed the development of dropsy as a side effect of this remedy. For nine years I have treated at the Charity Hospital, a large number of metal gilders (gold workers) suffering from mercurial tremor, sometimes with salivation, and I haven't seen a single case of dropsy, with coagulable urine, crop up at the same time as the tremor or following it." Now for the footnotes provoked by that terse paragraph which examines the historical point of view, as well as contributing his own observations.

"After examining the urine of four patients with mercurial salivation, Wells, (his observations were the most suggestive of a relationship) having found that the urine of three of the patients contained albumin (he) observed next the urine of six other persons suffering from venereal diseases, before they had taken any mercury. With five (of these controls) the urine contained no albumin, the urine of the sixth showed only traces. After two weeks of salivation the quantity of albumin had increased in three of the patients...Wells adds that other patients who were under treatment in his care for dropsies with coagulable urine had previously undergone mercurial treatments; and he concluded from these facts that mercury, administered in a high dose can cause the excretion of albumin in the urine and dropsy." Rayer quotes Wells very accurately but the exact wording of Wells' conclusion is, "It appears, therefore, from what has been said upon this part of my subject, that urine containing a considerable quantity of serum must occur very rarely, if at all, in any disease in this country, except dropsy, and that induced by mercury."

Continuing in this same footnote Rayer quotes Balackwell (Both Wells and Blackall reported their findings of dropsy and coagulable urine but without any reference to kidney disease before Bright's observations).. "Blackall reports four cases of dropsy with coagulable urine caused by mercury in high dosage." Dr. Christison also is quoted as citing a single case, "tending to prove that the effect of mercury … has some influence on the development of granular degeneration of the kidneys."

The references cited by Rayer would seem to be very suggestive that mercury could produce cogulable urine and perhaps even dropsy, but then as the final paragraph in this same footnote, as a sort of *coup de grace* to the argument, Rayer contributes his own study, "In 1835 I examined with Dr. Desir, at the Veneriens Hospital, the urine of 133 patients of whom 104 had early venereal symptoms, and 27 with symptoms developing later; 92 were submitted to external treatments (emollients, cauterizations, rubefacients etc); 41 used mercury (solution of cyanide of mercury, Sedillot pills, mercury rubs, cinnabar fumigations, etc) All these urines were tested with both heat and Nitric acid. Only two produced a light clot: one was from a corpulent woman, suffering from leukorrhea, with ulcerations on the cervix; the other had been a man infected with blennorrhea (gonorrhea) and orchitis: <u>so, in one of these cases, the albumin probably came from</u>

the secretions realated to the leukorrhea, and in the other by that of the blennorrhnea, which mixed with the urine at the time of his voiding." Such observations from 133 patients treated vigorously with mercurial preparations and not a single case of coagulable urine or dropsy (except for the two questionable cases that have been given a very acceptable explanation as to why their urines were slightly coagulable) probably gives an authoritative French answer to the relationship of the effect of mercury and coagulable urine, the examples from the prior literature not withstanding.

These are just a few representative examples of Rayer's use of footnotes in his chapter Nephrite Albumineuse from the *Traite des Maladies des Reins*. They confirm his comprehensive knowledge of the then extant literature, accurately citing various authors and contributors to the field, his penchant to speak his mind, both critically and with praise on the various prior author as well as contributing in the footnote data and observations of his own. Rayer's footnotes, as well as the other authors cited, provide a personal running commentary to the otherwise dry and pedantic text that often appears above them.

Summary

The use of footnotes varied among the authors who preceded Richard Bright as well as those who followed him in confirming and establishing the clinical entity of Bright's Disease. Richard Bright who gathered together the clinical and pathological findings to convincingly establish the kidney as the underlying pivotal factor in the explanation of coagulable urine and dropsy, eschewed the use of footnotes. Perhaps this was because he didn't feel his text needed the added spice of footnotes to make his points or that the suggestive but confusing observations of prior authors could be ignored. Certainly Bright didn't feel the compunction or academic need to garnish the text with exhaustive search of the literature. Was this a deliberate attempt to ignore the prior attempts to relate dropsy with coagulable urine to underlying kidney pathology or was it due to lack of a thorough literature search? Certainly John Blackall preceeding Bright, documents in footnotes a plethora of pertinent previous observations.

Richard Bright did acknowledge that his observations were "in a great degree in accordance with what has been laid down by Dr. Blackall in his most valuable treatise." But this was not in a footnote. William Wells writing in 1812, found no need to employ footnotes, writing in a flowing narrative style, oblivious of prior observations in the field and willing to forego the opportunity to challenge his text with harping or explanatory footnotes. Thomas Addison, a younger colleague and contributor of patients to Bright's *Case Reports* likewise found no need to use footnotes in his later publication of 1855 in *Disease of the Supra-renal Capsule.*

Ancient and Renaissance texts for the most part presented themselves in a grand narrative tradition without footnotes to clutter up the page and divert the reader. Perhaps writers like Bright, Wells, and Addison, while writing in the nineteenth century, deliberately chose their style to match there forebears, rather than join the crowd that followed the Enlightenment's innovation which saw footnotes proliferate. Gibbon in the *History of the Decline and fall of the Roman Empire,* Pierre Bayle in his *Historical and Critical Dictionary,* and Alexander Pope, peppering satirical footnotes in his *Variorum Dunciad* are examples of authors who used footnotes in a variety of ways that became popular in the Enlightenment. Rayer and Christison in their medical texts seemed to have joined this later club that used footnotes as an alternative text that competed with and acted as counterpoint to the text above it, vying for attention.

Christison and Rayer, who enthusiastically supported and extended the findings of Bright used footnotes not only to review the prior attempts to relate dropsy and coagulable urine to renal disease, but employed them as an equally important subtext to present even more interesting information than in the dry monotonous text above the ever running inventive, informative and discursive footnotes. The comparison of healthy and uremic urine and blood with respect to chemical analysis presented by Christison and the discussion of the naming of the disease by Rayer, all in footnotes, were worthy of separate articles in themselves. They are examples of footnotes being used as an alternative running battle with the text. Certainly a text such as Bright or Addison reads along effortlessly rather than fighting ones way through the footnoted obstacle course of Rayer or Christison. For those who can fathom up incisive original material in the form of uninterrupted discourses such as Bright and Addison, the footnote are an unwanted obstacles.

Robert Christison in his *Granular Degeneration,* discussing whether liver disease could be responsible for coagulable urine, justifies the use of footnotes forthrightly, "It would greatly perplex the reader if I entered in the text a full examination of the various facts and statements which have lately been put forward by others in contradistinction to the general principals laid down above. But it may be right to admit more particularly to the question in a note" (ie, a footnote). Alternatively he justified the use of footnotes "in order not to interrupt the train of statement given above (in the text)." Christison sees the footnote as a place to relegate disputed information, arguments pro and con, minutiae, and other controversial material so that it doesn't interrupt the flow of the text and perplex the reader. In this fashion the text is freed of difficult or extraneous material that allows the reader easy sailing in the text and allows only the adventurous to grapple with the footnotes.

Still footnotes represent valuable information and referenced material that allows further study by the reader. Anthony Grafton in *The Footnote* * *a curious history* tells the story of the youthful Harry Belafonte, "who in his early reading of W. E. B. DuBois, relates, 'I discovered that at the end of some sentences there was a number, and if you looked at the foot of the page the reference was to what it was all about—what source Du Bois gleamed his information from.' " Footnotes first inspired the young West Indian sailor to read critically."

Chapter Three

The Urinalysis as a Factor in the Establishment of the Clinical Entity Of Bright's Disease in the Early 19th Century

Summary: The study of the development and understanding of urinalysis as a tool in the diagnosis and management of renal disease in the early 19th Century, 1812-1840, is used as a marker for the recognition and reception of Richard Bright's momentous correlation of coaguable urine, dropsy and pathological identification of renal disease. The Animal Chemists, Berzelius, Prout, Bostock and Rees making strides in the analysis of urine are seen as out distancing the clinicians, Bright, Christison, Osborne, and Rayer who were unable to incorporate the findings of the Animal Chemists into bed side medicine .The clinicians, especially Bright encouraged the Animal Chemists to evaluate the usefulness of their findings as related to the care and management of patients. The examination of the urine from the early 19th Century is compared to the urinalysis of today.

The importance of the urine for diagnosis and treatment of diseases has an ancient and glorious past The definition of a Nephrologist could be considered as one who practices medicine but who also who looks at the urine. The Sumerian and Babylonian physicians according to Homer Smith in *De Urina,* gave attention to its color, consistency and frothiness. Galen praised Hippocratic medicine for their observation of the urine. Uroscopy in the Middle Ages became a fine art with the practice of divination.   Alchemy contributed   by identifying the salts of ammonia, ammonium chloride and ammonium sulfate as well as the identification of phosphorous by the alchemist Brandt in Hamburg in 1669. Sugar had been identified in the urine by the ancients and rediscovered by Thomas Willis, as recorded in his publication on the brain in 1664. Urea was first recovered in an impure form by Von Rouelle. Hermann Boerhaave, physician and chemist at Leyden is also given credit, describing it as a soapy material, soluable in alcohol and forming crystals, and on distillation producing a volatile alkaline material, ammonia. Latter Fourcroy and Vauquelin developed a more quantitative analysis of the substance they called uree.

Protein had been described in the urine before Richard Bright's salient linking of a) coagulable urine" when exposed to heat of a candle in a spoon", b) dropsy, and c) detailed findings at autopsy of abnormalities of the kidneys in 1827. William Cruikshank, reported albumin in diabetic patients as early as 1798. William Charles Wells, born in South Carolina who returned to England because of British sympathy during the American Revolutionary War, described as many as seventy eight patients with coaguable urine and dropsy, but did not correlate these findings with pathological studies and so missed out on defining the clinical syndrome of renal disease. Dr. John Blackall of St. Bartholomew's Hospital in London was recognized by Richard Bright in 1827 in the introduction of this *Case Reports* as having recognized coagulable urine and renal damage.

However the medical doctors who examined the urine in the early 19th century, while describing the urine grossly, as the uroscopists had done and carefully noting the presence or absence of coagulable urine; ie, protein, and measuring its Specific Gravity or density did little else to employ urinalysis in the evaluation of their patients. This was primarily due to the fact that while the microscope had been invented two hundred years earlier by Leewenhook, the unavailability of achromatic lenses made it difficult to view red and white cells, casts, crystals and other elements in the urine. (The same limitation, plus the unavailability of tissue micotomes to provide adequate thin sections of tissue, applied to the evaluation of tissue section of the kidney.) Not until Pierre Rayer's impressive Atlas of renal diseases in 1838 were such elements of the urine beautifully recorded. Even then urinalysis consisted primarily of determination of protein and Specific Gravity. Apparently these physicians of the early 19th Century had not respected the admonition of a leading renal physiologist of the 20th Century, Homer Smith. "Gather together all the lab hydrometers and carry them to the highest point in the hospital and drop them off', eliminating this test in urinalysis, since Homer Smith pointed out that the kidney doesn't process density but rather osmolality. (The physicians of the 21 Century have not gotten this message either, since this ancient analysis appears on every urinalysis result today)

The performance of urinalysis at the beginning of the 19th century was in the hands of the Animal Chemists, those who studied the chemical nature of living matter, such as J.J. Berzelius, in Sweden, John Bostock, William Prout, and George Owen Reese in England. Working with the background studies of the Ancients, the Uroscopist, and the French chemists Forcrcroy and Vauquelin, among others, a urinalysis was mostly a chemical analysis affair, rather than a urinalysis in the modern sense of a microscopic examination of the urine or a dip stick report. This in spite of the momentous discovery of Richard Bright using urine protein as a critical component of trilogy that linked dropsy with pathological confirmation. Bright frequently recorded the volume of the urine produced, describing the urine as dingy, or its odor as ammoniacial, or its appearance as brown and turbid with deposits of brown sediment or waxing over the appearance of the precipitate, "The coagulation is in different degrees: it likewise differs somewhat in its character: most commonly when the urine has been exposed to the heat of a candle in a spoon, before it rises quite to the boiling point it becomes clouded, sometimes simply opalescent, at other times almost like milk beginning at the edges of the spoon and quickly meeting in the middle, etc" His physician colleagues, animal chemists, John Bostock and others provided crude but critical chemical analysis. It was not until Pierre Rayer's *Traite des Maladies des Reins* and especially the Atlas that preceded its publication in 1839, twelve years after Bright's *Case Reports*, that the urine was being examined under the microscopic, with the recording of red cells and casts and crystals, in a fashion similar to a modern urinalysis.

J.J.Berzelius, Animal Chemist

In 1813 J.J. Berzelius a physician but who became primarily a chemist studying the basis composition of matter and using the blow pipe as an instrument for mineral analysis, published a Volume entitled, *A View of the Progress and Present State of Animal Chemistry*, the last 20 pages devoted to the study of the urine. Earlier parts of this volume are devoted to the current knowledge of the chemistry of gastric juice, nervous system tissue, muscle and connective tissue, hair, etc. Berzelius begins by noting that urine "has undergone more chemical examination than that of any other animal matter." He reviews Van Helmont's treatise on the stone, the discovery of phosphorous in the urine by Brandt and Kunkel, the work of Boerhaave, the analysis of the "younger Rouelle's" in characterizing a saponaceous extract, latter identified as urea by Cruikshank and later by Fourcroy and Vauquelin. He then lists his contribution to the animal chemistry of the urine, identifying sulphuric and phosphoric acid, separating colorless crystals of urea. He quotes the studies of Fourcroy and Vauquelin on the identification of uric acid in the excrements of birds from the South seas, called Guano, and describes the latter's finding a uric acid stone from the bladder of a tortoise, "from which it appears at man is not the only animal in whose body this acid is generated." He goes on to discuss stone formation and considers diet in the control of uric acid stones, but comes to the conclusion that "it is often impossible to diminish the acid of the urine by the use of alkali in those that suffer from an excess of uric acid." He concludes," For my part, I have endeavoured to unite chemical and anatomical researches in the pursuit of one common object, in order thus to give to the investigation of the Animal Chemist, a determined and scientific tendency, and to his efforts, a physiological view. And I foresee, with pleasure, that, when more able men than myself shall hereafter occupy themselves with researches in Animal Chemistry, in the same manner as I have done, this interesting Science will acquire a degree of perfection, which, at present, we not only do not expect, but scarcely even venture to hope."

In recording his characterization of urine, he indicates "I have taken up the investigation of this subject, and have obtained results which have escaped the attention of my predecessors." Berzelius continues, "I found in the urine a considerable quantity of sulphuric and phosphoric acid, the former of which is not discernible in the blood, and the latter only in a very minute quantity." He also comments, "the portion of the earthy and alkaline salts (oxides of a metal of the group of which calcium and magnesium belong), which the urine contains, is also very considerable whereas in the blood it is but small."

He discusses the mucus of the bladder, "always partly suspended, and partly dissolved ......in combination with the uric acid." Going on to discuss urea, "The urea which my predecessors had described, I found to be a composition of urea, properly so called, and several deliquescent substances, devoid of colour, and forming distinct prismatic crystals like nitre (potassium nitrate)" From this description, the isolation of urea must have been very pure. He also finds, "a mineral substance, which had been overlooked by them, vis, silica." The blow-torch that Berzelius developed was very adapt at detecting small quantities of minerals such as silica.

Berzelius a year earlier in 1812, in Medico- Chirurigical Transactions, Vol. 3 recorded a remarkable complete and accurate analysis of the urine based on the above analysis:

> Water 933.00 parts by weight
> Urea 30.10
> Potassium Sulphate 3.71
> Sodium Sulphate 3.16
> Sodium Phosphate 2.94
> Sodium Chloride4.45
> Ammonium Phosphate 1.65
> Ammonium Phosphate 1.50
> Lactic acid; ammonium lactuate; Alcohol-soluble
> and alcohol-insoluble Animal matter 17.14
> Earthy phosphates; calcium fluoride 1.00
> Uric Acid 1.00
> Mucus of the bladder 0.32

Silex (silica) 0.03

1000.00

Urea is determined to be the major component of the urine, and considering the daily urine volume to be one liter, a reasonable estimate, with the 30 gm   of urea which would   correlate with a protein intake of ninety to one hundred grams. The amount of sodium, considering the three sodium salts, would amount to about four grams of sodium or 70 mEq. and would be a reasonable   estimate of sodium intake. Potassium from the potassium sulphate would represent only 1.8 grams which would be rather low. Lactic acid is an unlikely substance in the urine. Uric acid of 1000 mg seems high, unless this sample was from and over producer of uric acid.   The Silex (silica) Brezelius explains as a contaminant of the water supply that appears in the urine.

Such a chemical analysis of the urine in 1812 represented a dramatic, if at times an imprecise estimate, that stood head and shoulders above the clinicians observation of the urine at the time, and represented a beginning for the understanding of renal disease.

William Prout, Animal Chemist in the Circle of Richard Bright

William Prout   was probably the most outstanding animal chemist in England, following the lead of Berzelius in developing atomic theory,   working eventually with Richard Bright. Prout prepared very pure crystals of urea and established the presence of the stong acid, Hydrochloric acid, as a component   of human gastric juice. With regard to the study of urinalysis, he published in 1825,   two years before Richard Bright's *Case Reports* entitled *"An inquiry into the nature and treatment of diabetes, calculus, and other affections of the urinary organs"* The author goes on to indicate the "importance of attending to the state of the urine in organic diseases of the kidney and bladder, and some practical rules for determining the nature of the disease from the sensible and chemical properties of that secretion." Following Berzelius a chemical approach is taken with a description of urea, lithic acid (uric acid) oxalic acid, carbonic acid and even Benzoic acid which was probably a methodological error. Prout had demonstrated that urine from Bright's patients had a reduced quantity of urea. He had also observed that phosphates in alkaline urine would precipitate and be re-dissolved on adding acid, unlike albumin. But the most striking aspect of this text was the Table of Test, Apparatus, etc., required in making Experiments on the Urine:

1. Perhaps the following list may not be deemed superfluous by some of my readers. <u>Litmus Paper</u>, blue and red; <u>Turmeric Paper</u>, By these all points connected with the asescency and alkalescency of the urine may be determined.

2. A <u>Watch Glass</u>, or what is better a thin platinum Vessel of the same shape, for detecting an excess of urea, evaporation, etc.

3. Two small Discs of Plate-glass for discriminating pus from mucus, according to Dr. Young's method. They are also useful for other purposes.

4. <u>A Bottle for determining the specific gravity</u> of urine. Or what is better, a small portable <u>hydromete</u>r, made by Tuther, 221, High Holborn, for that purpose, and which is sufficiently

accurate for practical use.

5.   A Blow-pipe, Forceps, etc, by which almost every experiment that can be required can be readily made on gravel or calculous matter, so as to lead to a knowledge of their nature.

6.   These, with one or two small test tubes, and small stoppered phials, containing solutions of pure ammonia, potash, and nitric acid can be readily packed in to a small portable case, or pocket-book, and will be sufficient, by the aid of a common taper or candle, to perform all the experiments on the urine, and urinary productions, that are commonly necessary in a practical point of view.

The modern Nephrologist who performs urinalysis is likely to recognize only three of the items from Prout's *Required* items in making *Experiments on the Urine: 1)* The Litmus paper, 2) a Bottle for determining the specific gravity, a portable hydrometer, and 3) the two small test tubes. The blow-pipe was an instrument developed and perfected by Berzelius, and as indicated by Prout was for analysis of minerals found in calculi, and would be today ordered as a separate determination in a lab devoted to stone analysis. Pus would be looked for under the microscope, but Prout following Berzelius recognized mucus as a major feature of the "urinalysis" and needed to differentiate it from pus, presumably by chemical means. Urea is not ordinarily a part of a urinalysis, but with this chemical perspective to urinalysis, became an important semi quantitative analysis of renal function, in that a reduction of urea in the urine, as well as a reduced specific gravity would be taken as evidenced of impaired renal function This will become more evident as we examine the studies of Christison and Rayer. Bright in his Gulstonian Lecture of 1833, acknowledges from the pen of Dr. Prout a work on urinary secretion, "a subject upon which we possess-----no more concise, accurate or more philosophic in character."

Richard Bright and the 1827 Reports of Medical Cases

Richard Bright's publication in 1827 *of Reports of Medical Cases Selected with a view of illustrating The Symptoms and Cure of Diseases by reference to Morbid Anatomy (Reports of Medical Cases) while* mentioning nothing about urinalysis or kidney disease, and falsely promises a cure, was a milestone event in establishing a clinical-pathological entity that linked pathological changes in the kidneys, dropsy with a clinical picture of complications of renal disease and proteinuria. The finding of coagulable urine when exposed to the "heat of a candle in a spoon" was not a new finding, having been observed by John Blackall and William Wells previously, but it was the linking of this with the clinical and pathological features that cemented a clinical-pathological entity. Otherwise Bright contributed little of note to the study of the urine himself. However he was omniscient enough to delegate these studies to his younger colleagues, among whom were Prout, Bostock, Babington and the medical student Mr. Treedy.

Bright's contribution to the study of the urine, except for the cogent observation of coaguable urine representing a critical part of the clinical-pathological entity of this newly characterized clinical, was primarily a descriptive record of the various characteristics of the precipitate formed when urine is heated. Bright was visually oriented as can be confirmed by the magnificent mezzotint lithographs that are the glory of *Case Reports*. From this volume Bright describes coagulation of the urine by heat stating, " The coagulation is in different degrees: before it rises quite to a boiling point it becomes clouded, sometimes simply opalescent, at other times almost milky, beginning at the edges of the spoon and quickly meeting in the middle. In a short time the coagulating particles break up into a flocculent or a curdled form, and the quantity of this flocculent matter varies from a quantity scarcely perceptible floating in the fluid, to so much as converts the whole into the appearance of curdled milk", etc, etc. He recognized " a great tendency to throw off the red particles of the blood by the kidneys, betrayed by various degrees of haematuria from the simple dingy colour of the urine, which is easily recognized; or the slight brown deposit;- to the completely bloody urine, when the whole appears to be little but blood, and when not infrequently a thick ropy deposit is found a the bottom of the vessel" This is a detailed meticulous description of the urine, but doesn't approach the findings of Berzelius fifteen years earlier or Prout's description of his equipment for *Tests, Apparatus etc, required in making Experiments on the Urine.*

John Bostock, George Owen Rees and the Animal Chemist in the Circle of Richard Bright

Bright delegated to John Bostock, MD the task of analyzing further the urines on many of the 23 cases that made up the Case Reports. In three letter, the first ten pages long Bostock details his findings more from the aspect of the animal chemists. The heading of the letters is *Observations on the Chemical properties of the Foregoing Cases*, dated Upper Bedford Place, April 24the 1824. He begins, "I propose in this letter to give you some account of the experiments which I have performed on the various specimens of morbid urine which I have received from you, for the purpose of illustrating your pathological observations." Bostock goes on to indicate he examined 28 specimens from a selection of Bright's cases, six from the patient Roderick, five from Plume, etc. He concludes that the Specific Gravity of the Urine is generally "reduced in dropsical that coagulates." This was a generally agreed upon observation of the followers of Bright, Christison and Rayer. The cause of this reduced SpG is considered as either: " 1) as natural urine in a state of dilution,2) as having a deficiency in the proportion of some of its ingredients; or, 3) together with this deficiency, as containing some extraneous substance." He concludes favoring the third possibility without and evidence to support "some extraneous substance." Bostock further studied the effect of bloodletting on SpG with indeterminate results.

He continues on to affirm that the albumin of dropsical urine and the whites of the egg are similar because their reaction with heat and various chemicals are identical. He considers the effect of "the presence of uncombined acid and alkali (pH) on the separation of the albumen, as produced by the application of heat. The next consideration is the relationship of the "in what quantity albumen exits, with what proportion it bears to the urea and salts." For this analysis acting as an animal chemist rather than the observational reports of Bright, Bostock evaporates the healthy urine to a thick extract, digests with alcohol to remove urea, and dissolves the residue with water, by which the greatest part of the salts was dissolved." By this method, Bostock confesses "I obtained results which although by no means perfectly accurate were sufficiently so for the object in view." He concluded, "supposing the whole to amount to 6 % of the weigh of the urine, it will give us 4% urea and 2% salts." Remarkably this roughly agrees with the early analysis of Berzelius quoted earlier above from 1812! He next planned to "inquire how far the composition of some of the specimens of (coaguable) urine differed with the above proportion." There was never a clear answer to this question, but he concludes, "the results of my experiments generally (indicate) that the quantity of albumen in the urine bore no exact relation to the total amount of its solid contents, or to that of the urea in particular." As far as this statement goes it can be considered a reasonable observation.

Bostock continues with a an apology, "I may appear to be encroaching upon your (Bright's) province if I offer any remarks upon the inferences which may be drawn from the presence of this albuminous matter in the urine; but as my remarks will principally refer to the chemical nature of the fluid, you will perhaps think them not altogether out of place." Here Bostock separates himself from Bright, in emphasizing that he is doing a chemical analysis, agreeing with my prior discussion that Bright's province was only the qualitative aspect of observing the urine. Bostock goes on to indicated that albuminuria might not always represent a "morbid state and may be produced by such a variety of circumstances, and many of them of so trifling a nature. In my own person I have very seldom found the fluid to be entirely free from it, and I have observed it to be increased to a considerable amount by the slightest causes.." Here Bostock for the first time indicated the existence of benign types of proteinuria. This was a subject Sir William Osler was to have more fully characterized in his 1892 section on Albuminuria in *The Principles and Practice of Medicine*, in1982

The second and third letter are briefer and Bostock began studying the blood and came to the conclusion, "We have here therefore, and example of the blood exhibiting a very great deficiency of albumin, at the same time that we observe the mode in which it passes off from the system by means of the kidney, while this organ has its appropriate office of secreting urea nearly suspended." Presumably this was a patient with renal failure ("kidney's secreting function nearly suspended"), and nephrotic syndrome (blood exhibiting a very great deficiency of albumin and the observing the mode in which it (albumin) passes off from the system by means of the kidney. Bostock identifies this patient as "Sarah Sutton 25 years old, a woman of intemperate habits attacked with anasarca about two months earlier and who has lately become the subject of ascites. The quantity of urine which she passes is very small., but she is at present improving under the employment of small bleedings and gentle diuretics. At some future time I shall report the progress and termination of this case."

In summary Bostock studies the effect of SpG of the urine under various conditions, identifies egg albumin and albuminuria as identical on the basis of chemical tests, identifies coaguable urine as albuminuria, attempts to relate albuminuria, urea and the solids of the urine, points out benign causes of albuminuria, including himself who may have this form of benign proteinuria, and describes the nephrotic syndrome with renal failure.

George Owen Rees followed Bostock, providing chemical correlations to the clinical findings of Bright. An adjoining two ward, on for males the other for females were set up to study the newly recognized disease. Rees wanted to bring simple chemical techniques to the clinical arena. He published a book using techniques of Berzelius, using his method of analysis of lithic (uric) acid in the urine and Prout's method for urea. He advocated the use of both heat and nitric acid of determining albumin in the urine, and to differentiate the precipitates of phosphate and albumin, since phosphates would dissolve in acid.

An epidemiological study for the present of coaguable urine on the wards of Guy's Hospital was initiated, and Bright reports that in 1832, My friends Dr. G. H. Barlow and Mr Tweedie understood to make for me a still more extensive experiment, extending to nearly 300 individuals, finding one in eleven decidedly affected with the disease." An additional 141 patients were studied later. "In this experiment, the proportion of cases considered albuminous amounted to above one in six." These rather high incidences of albuminuria in the general hospital population could represent an error in the method of demonstrating albuminuria or perhaps the influence of renal toxicity from the wide spread use of mercury.

Robert Christison "The Bright of Scotland"

Sir Robert Christison was a Scotchman from Edinburgh, several years behind Richard Bright at the Edinburgh Medical School. He was Bright's earliest and most enthusiastic follower, recognizing and proselytizing the existence of renal disease, as Variety of Dropsy which Depends on Kidney Disease promulgated by the Guy's Hospital physician. Christison writes in his *Observation on the Variety of Dropsy which Depends on Kidney Disease*, just two years after Bright's *Case Reports*, "no other physician has publicly noticed his discovery or endeavored to confirm or extend his statement that dropsy appears to originate in organic derangement of the kidney and is one of the frequent varieties of this disease." In this 1829 publication he presented seven cases that mirrored Bright's finding of dropsy in the present of coaguable urine and evidence of renal involvement. And what about the examination of the urine? In addition to the presence of proteinuria and measurement of specific gravity, Christison made significant progress in comparing "normal " urine with that of his patients as can be seen from the following table:

Control Pt Rt. Irving
Patient: J.Thompson
Volume   110 oz   35oz
                30 oz

SpG	1029	1013.4
	1009.1	
Solids	67.7/1000	29.8/1000
	22.8/1000	
Urea/animal	Acetate	
	55.2/1000	20.4/1000
	16.9/1000	
Alkaline Murates		
Sulfate/Phosphates	11.1/100	3.7/1000
	3.3/1000	
Earthy Phosphates 1.0/1000		inappreciable
inappreciable		
Vesical mucous	0.4	-------

Albumin	---------	5.1/10000
1.5/1000		

This data has been obtained primarily from footnotes of Christison's text where the details of examination of the urine are recorded. The conclusions are clear that urine volume, SpG, solids, and phosphates are reduced with the presence of albumin in the urine in the patients he described as compare with the control.

The first case is Robert Irving, an out-pensioner of Chelsea Hospital, robust, short stature, presenting with edema and enlargement of abdomen, subject to general exposure of vicissitudes of temperature at his employment as a porter in a butcher shop. He had a battered dissipated appearance allowing he had led a very intemperate life. (alcohol and exposure to cold were considered etiological factors in the disease) Four ounces of urine produced a copious flocculent precipitate with ebullition (bubbles) The above urine studies were taken during the course of a six month hospitalization characterized by increasing edema, dysentery, anorexia, headache and dimness of vision, cough, respiratory symptoms, during which the urine urea, solids, and specific gravity were measured on a number of occasions. The patient's medication were legion: Squill, Supertartrate of Potassium, Mercury, Blisters to the head, leaches, Phlebotomy,etc. Remarkably the patient was able to be dismissed, but returned and died within several days. Post showed small, hard, pale, scabrous granular kidnies.(Christison's spelling).

The exact meaning of some of the above headings, urea/ animal acetates, alkaline murates, earthy phosphates, etc may be in doubt, but this is the first attempt to perform a series of tests on the urine of patients with Bright's disease and compare them with control urine. In addition Christison prepares a correlation of SpG and Solids:

SpG :
1020   ------   68 Solids/1000
1024.8 ------   81Solids/1000
1030.4 ------   102 Solids/1000

More detailed correlations of SpG and Solids were to be presented by Rayer. In addition for the first time in clinical renal medicine a fairly reasonable attempt was made to measure the urea content in the blood in his second patient, Frances Magee. . Bostock had measured the urea concentration in the hydrocephalic fluid on one of Brights's patients. Christison reports: One ounce of the blood of Magee was heated in a vapor bath, the red granular mass is taken up with distilled water, filtered, evaporated to dryness, extracted with alcohol, evaporated in a watch glass, and then on the addition of a few drops of nitric acid there immediately appeared fine grayish red flaky crystals of a pearly luster—"these evidently were scales of nitrate of urea!" Urea had never been demonstrated in normal patients or convincingly in renal disease, so that any at all would represent an excessive amount.

In the later 1839 volume, *On Granular Degeneration of the Kidneys and its Connection with Dropsy, Inflammations, and other Diseases,* Christison would present additional considerations of the evaluation of the urine. In a long footnote on page 21 of this volume, Christison, in discussing the the nature of the precipitation of albumin with heat, he indicates that, " The best way of operating is with a tube about a third of an inch inch in diameter – A spoon, which may be used, is a clumsy substitute which will not show the nice degree of coagulability. (This in spite if Bright's directions to observe "the coagulation in different degrees—when the urine has been exposed to the heat of a candle in a <u>spoon</u>") Christison does to try to quantitate the amount of protein present: " 1. Gelatin by heat, 2 Very strong coagulability, 3. Strongly coaguable, 4 Moderately coaguable, 5. Feelby coagulable, 6. Hazy by heat." Then Christison comments on a procedure all current nephrologist perform by instinct or observation of others, " In appreciating the least degree of impregnation (of the protein precipitate), it is convenient <u>to heat only the upper half of the fluid in the tube.</u>" Now that was something Bright missed.

In addition to confirming Bright's finding with regard to renal disease as being a factor in many cases of dropsy, Christison laid out hope of potential reversibility of the condition since several of his cases improved or recovered. Bright speculated that recovery was possible but never demonstrated this in his cases. Christison was impatient with his fellow practitioners in not recognizing Bright's findings, " which were received at first with coldness by his brethren, It was said that such cases as he described had been seen only in Guy's Hospital, and in the scum alone of the London population—(but) by and by, Bright's disease was recognized in all stations of life, by all medical men, and only in too great abundance."

Jonathan Osborne of Dublin

Jonathan Osborne of Dublin, Physician to Sir Patrick Dun's and Mercer Hospital closely followed Christison's report with a series of 23 cases of his own following Bright's criteria for renal disease. Osborne's particular take on the etiology of Bright's disease was the concept of suppressed perspiration and recommended measures to improve this situation, such as warm baths With regard to evaluation of the urine, he had one "fixed rule"– the urine was to be examined before breakfast and only after is had cooled. Some doctors today continue to advise their patients to follow just such a procedure. Osborne also made comments on the differentiating oxalates from phosphate in the urine: the former in acid urine produce a cloudy appearance with heat but the urine becoming clear near the boiling point, phosphates continue to present as a cloud when boiling is approached. (Prout had shown earlier that adding acid to alkaline urine would dissolve precipitates of phosphates.)

Pierre Rayer Traite des Maladies des Reins Definitive Renal Textbook of Early19th Century

Gabriel Richet's *From Bright's Disease to Modern Nephrology: Pierre Rqyer's Innovative Method of Clinical Investigation* summaries the contribution of Pierre Rayer's contribution to renal studies in France. Rayer introduced the works of Bright, Christison and Osborne to Paris. His two volume *Traite des Maladies des Reins et des Alterations de la Secretion Urirnaire,* a two volume work with over 2000 pages was published in 1840. Its accompanying large atlas of drawings of renal abnormalities published in 1838, contributed to further evaluation of study of the urine in renal disease. Described in detail in the first volume, under the title of *Prolegomena* is a preliminary evalution of methods It compares to a physiology text of today, in discussing the findings with out reference to clinical consideration. An historical review is followed a consideration of many of the factors previously considered by the English School of physicians,ie: SpG, Urea, *ac. urique* (uric acid), phosphates, alkalinity, mucus, *nuages sedimens* (cloudy sediment), albumin, and in addition using a microscope for the first time in renal evaluation red blood cells (glob sang) pus, fatty and oily material. There are appended to the first volume six plates of detailed microscopic drawings, Hexagonal crystals of Cysteine, crystals of Quinine, ammonium phosphate, Hippuric acid (ac. de cheval), red blood cells, sperm and globules of fat (*globules du lait*) These microscopic drawings were possible because of the development of Charles Louis Chevalier who perfected an achromatic lens for the microscope. There is a detailed chart relating SpG to Solids, much improved over the few values noted previously by Christison. He confirmed the English School's finding of reduced SpG in the urine of chronic *Nephrite Albumineuse* (Rayer's term for Bright's Disease) because of the reduction of urea and salts counter acting the presence of albumin. Rayer recognized the presence of albumin in some cases of pregnany. He established suppurative pyelonephritis. The last chapter of the second volume of the Traite consists of over 100 pages of historical bibliography documenting in comprehensive fashion the literature on kidney disease up until 1840.

An examination of the chapter on *Nephrite Albumineuse* in the second volume of Rayer after a long introduction, includes 24 cases which are described in detail with clinical descriptions, lavish discussions of treatments (bloodletting, leaches, horseradish tea, donkey milk, couch-grass tea, gamboges, cream of tartar, colchicum tea, warm baths, aromatic fumigation, steam baths, etc). There is very little attention to the examination of the urine, however. There are no microscopic examination, as were reported in the first volume, rarely measurement of SpG. Clearly the examination of the urine played no or little role in the diagnosis or management of the clinical condition. Reviewing the attention Rayer gave to the urine reveals : Case 1, Madam C. Spanish, very strong constitution, exposed o cold and dampness, urine became reddish and formed abundant sediment, generalized swelling, her urine contained a strong proportion of albumin, couch-grass tea, an impressive failure made bleeding necessary, horseradish half ounce in a pint of water, urine became more abundant, progressively less murky, less tinged with blood and finally less albuminous and the dropsy disappeared completely, " After a cure of the anasarca, Madame Continued for a while the use of donkey milk" No reoccurrence. Case 2, M.Triqueneaux: urine color-natural, deposit of mucous and uric acid, later the urine described as citrine, considerable precipitate with nitric acid and heat, Case 7: Anne Filiat- Nitric acid produced mild cloudiness, but no flakes(shades of Bright's description), "urine pale without sediment limpid, neutral on the test paper, nitric acid doesn't produce the slightest clouds, but heat clouds a bit, its transparency to the point of <u>making it look like water from the Seine during the rainy season</u>", Case 16 P. Tessier by accident examination of the urine omitted! etc. The sophistication shown in the first volume of the *Traite* is not carried through to the clinical level. Rayer does advise against use of bladder urine to evaluate proteinuria (several of Bright's cases used post mortem bladder urine where the initial urine had not obtained)

Conclusion

The development of urinalysis in the first half of the 19th Century, 1812-1840. has been considered. Urinalysis was primarily the province of the Animal Chemists, using crude, but ever increasing sophisticated methods. Richard Bright's genius was in culling a single test on the urine, the coaguablity of urine, and making it a touch stone for defining a clinical-pathological entity. Renal calculi had been studied, beginning a hundred years earlier by Rev. Stephen Hales, followed by Scheele on uric acid stones, and then Fourcry, Wallaston and Marcet, leading to much information for the Animal Chemists Richard Bright and his followers 1827 through 1840 supported and tried to use the newer information from the Animal Chemists, but their clinical decisions were primarily concerned by the finding of coaguable urine, indicating albuminuria and perhaps following SpG. The unavailability of the microscope and the inexactness and labor intensiveness of the chemical methods of the Animal Chemists made their procedures difficult to apply at the bed side. Also the absence of physiological consideration such as renal function and nitrogen metabolism made the study of the urine as a hand maiden of clinical diagnosis cumbersome and impractical. Pierre Rayer in the introductory discussion of his Traite correctly indicated however:" *A la verite, on s'etait, pour ainsi dire, ferme d'avance de chemin des observations fruitueuses, et ote les moyens de penetrer avant dans le diagnostic et le traitement des maladies renales, en laissant dans l'ombre les alterations de la secretion urinaire* " (In truth, not to consider the alterations in urinary secretion is to close oneself off from fruitful observation on penetrating into the diagnosis and treatment of renal disease.) Rayer as noted above addressed these issues in his introductory *Prolegemena* but in applying these consideration to clinical management of patients as outlined in the chapter *Nephrite Albumineuse,* he was no further advanced than Bright. This is nothing new, since clinical medicine is always behind the basic science supporting it. This is like political arguments and speech, the promises of the orator far out weight the actual deliver of the message. Christison is given high marks for trying to apply the methods of the Animal Chemists to the analysis of the urine and to Bright and Rayer I would give even higher accolades for fostering and promulgating the investigation of the Animal chemists.

When a physician reviews a report of a urinalysis, or a nephrologist actually examines the urine himself, Albumin and SpG stand out as shads from the early 19th century. Earthy phosphates, alkaline murate, and vesical mucous, are no longer recognized in the report Is it time to eliminate the ancient test for SpG, recommended along with the blow pipe, the watch glass and the Turmeric paper from the kit of William Prout and follow Homer Smith and chuck out the hydrometers from the highest towers of our hospitals?

Chapter Four

The Animal Chemists in the Circle of Richard Bright

A physician in 1827 who would have examined a copy of the recently published *Reports of Medical Cases selected with a view of illustrating The Symptoms and Cure of Diseases by a reference to Morbid Anatomy* would have found a landmark publication by Richard Bright of Guys Hospital in London,England. Here would be defined a renal disease as a combination of dropsy, i.e. edema, coagulable urine, and shrunken granular kidneys at autopsy. However there were very little quantitative or chemical features that characterized this trilogy. Bright was a clinician trained to observe and record events carefully. The coagulable urine or proteinuria was observed as a "coagulation in different degrees when urine was exposed to the heat of a candle in a spoon." There was no chemical or quantative measurement of the albumin. The urine was never examined under a microscope, and chemical and quantitative measurements of urine or blood for urea nitrogen, creatinine, or electrolytes were unknown at that time. However Bright did encourage a handful of physician colleagues to amplify and pursue the chemical and physical properties of the blood, urine and other fluids in these patients with the newly defined trilogy of renal disease.

These physicians at Guys Hospital came to specialize in the newly blossoming study of the chemical nature of products of animals including humans, analyzing bile, stomach contents, blood and urine as well as kidney stones. Some of the physicians learned their trade as an apprentice to the apothecary of Guys Hospital. Others were influenced by the early chemists on the Continent. Their efforts were to describe and learn more about the illnesses they found on the wards of the Guys Hospital, using chemical methods to amplify and expand their understanding of disease processes, leading to possible treatment as well. These physicians were called Animal Chemists, and this paper is directed to the understanding and characterizing these Animal Chemists in the circle of Richard Bright.

Animal Chemists

Who were these Animal Chemists? The most famous and productive were J.J. Berzelius in Sweden and J.von Liebig in Germany. In England, working at Guys Hospital with Bright were Alexander Marcet, Johns Bostek, William Prout, George Owen Reese, Benjamin Babington, G.H.Barlow and Mr. Tweedie, a medical student, as well as others. In France the Animal Chemists such as Antoine Francois de Fourcroy and L. N. Vauquelin jointly published papers on urine, tears, blood and bile and other animal fluids. Also in France J. B. A. Dumas contributed to animal and plant chemistry. Perhaps the outstanding chemists of the early nineteenth century were J. J. Berzelius in Sweden and Justin von Liebig in Germany. These two chemists provided basic analysis of composition and structure of chemical compounds that supported the Animal Chemists of the Continent and England.

Renal Function

What was known concerning renal function at the time of Bright's observations on the correlation of protein in the urine, dropsy and contracted kidneys? That the kidneys made urine was a given. Homer W. Smith in his article De Urina quotes the Danish writer Isak Dinesen in her Seven Gothic Tales, " What is man, when you come to think upon him, but a minutely set, ingenious machine for turning, with infinite artfulness, the red wine of Shiraz into urine?" Urine has been advocated as a treatment of disease as well as playing a role in diagnosis since antiquity . Uroscopy, the practice of holding the urine up in a specially shaped flask served a diagnostic function during the Middle Ages.

Urea

Urea was first characterized in a crude preparation by Hilaire Marin Rouelle (1718-1779) in 1773 by obtaining an alcoholic extract of the residue of evaporated urine from both human and animal sources. He called it *matiere savonneuse* or soapy material and described how on heating it contained more than half its weight of ammonia. Hermann Boerhaave (1668-1738) physician and chemist at Leyden should be given prior credit in his "Elementa Cheniae" published in 1732. This material was obtained by heating urine to 200 degrees, washing the residue in water, producing crystals of what he called "native salt of urine" Fourcroy and Vauquelin prepared a purer preparation and were the first to call this material uree. In 1802 they jointly published a paper on the chemistry and compositions of urine. Fourcroy and Vauquelin were the first to analyse the urine of birds and reptiles and found uric acid rather than urea.

They described uric acid as well as a number of mineral salts such as sodium and ammonium phosphates. They also claimed to have found benzoic acid but this could not be confirmed by the Swedish chemist Berzelius who also prepared urea by precipitating with oxalate. This benzoic acid was probably hippuric acid, a similar compound that contains nitrogen. Fourcroy and Vauquelin also showed that the decomposition products of urea contained a very high proportion of azote (nitrogen) and considered that the physiological function of the kidneys was the removal azote from the body. Chemistry and Physiology were not capable of evaluating this suggestion at that time. Berzelius in 1812analysed urine and found the following proportions :

Water	933.0 parts by weight
Urea	30.1 ' ' '
Sodium chloride	4.5 " " "
Potassium sulphate	3.7 ' " "

The relative proportions of these substances so estimated indicated that urea was the most abundant substance in urine except for water.

Proteinuria

Richard Bright was not the first to report protein in the urine. William Cruikshank, Apothecary to the Army Hospital at Woolwich had reported albumin in diabetic patients as early as 1798. He is also is reported by J. Rollo in An Account of Two Cases of the Diabetes Melletitus, 1797, to have isolated urea with Nitric Acid., and this was recognized by Fourcroy, who claimed priority, however. William Charles Wells, who was born in South Carolina but returned to England because of British sympathy during the American Revolutionary War, described as many as seventy eight patients with coagulable urine and dropsy, but did not correlate this with careful pathological studies. Dr. John Blackall of St. Bartholomew's Hospital also recognized coagulable urine and renal damage and was recognized by Richard Bright in the 1827 introduction of <u>Case Reports,</u> "The observations which I have made respecting the condition of the urine in dropsy, are in a great degree in accordance with what has been laid down by Dr. Blackall in his most valuable treatise."

William Prout and the Measurement of Urea in the Urine

William Prout one of the animal chemists associated with Richard Bright in London, emphasizing purity of his reagents, was one of the first to obtain fairly good samples of crystalline urea. His laborious method is describe by Noel C. Coley in <u>From Animal Chemistry to Biochemistry,</u> "Fresh urine was first evaporated to the consistency of a syrup and after cooling pure concentrated nitric acid was added until the whole had turned to a dark crystalline mass. These crystals were washed with cold distilled water and a solution of sodium or potassium carbonate was added to neutralize the nitric acid. The solution so formed was evaporated until it would crystallize to form sodium or potassium nitrate crystals and a solution containing impure urea. The crystals were filtered off and the solution was then boiled with animal charcoal in order to decolourise it. The mixture was again filtered, evaporated to half bulk and allowed to crystallize. These crystals, which were impure urea, were then filtered off and dissolved in boiling alcohol. After filtering the hot solution so formed the urea was allowed to crystallize from it in four sided, transparent crystals of fair purity." All that for some crystals of "fair" purity, which I supposed were weighed to determine the quantity present. Such tedious analyses contributed to the slow progress the Animal Chemists had in promulgating their art.

Prout is probably best know for his theory that atomic weights of elements were multiples of the atomic weight of hydrogen. He also proposed for the first time the division of food into sugar, fats and proteins. This appeared in the Philosophical Transactions of 1827,"....the principal elementary matters employed by man and the more perfect animals, might be reduced to three great classes, namely the saccharine, the oily and the albuminous."

That there was urea in the urine and in relatively large quantity was established by the intensive and convoluted analyses of Berzelius, Prout and others, but what was the relationship of urea to the kidney? Was urea made by the kidney and/or excreted by the kidney? In 1823 Dumas and Prevost addressed the matter and performed a critical study. The kidneys of an animal were removed and the urea in the blood often difficult to find in normal animals was found in large quantity. This strongly suggested that urea was made elsewhere than in the kidney, which was responsible for the elimination of urea alone.

Friedrick Wohler and the Production of Urea from Inorganic Sources

In 1828, the year after Richard Bright described the clinical-pathological entity of the renal disease that bears his name, Friedrick Wohler working with von Leibig demonstrate that a product of animal chemistry, urea, could be produced in the laboratory from the inorganic source, ammonium cyanate. While Wohler did not claim that this was a blow against Vitalism, the doctrine that some vital force had to be operative in the production of products from animal chemistry, others have considered it so. Wohler only claimed that a rearrangement had taken place; ie: NH4CNO----NH2CONH2,ammonium cyanate to urea.

Animal Chemist Alexander Marcet

With this background the role of the Animal Chemists around Richard Bright can be introduced. Alexander Marcet was a chemistry teacher of Richard Bright. Marcet was Swiss and was familiar with many of the European Animal Chemists including Berzelius. It was Marcet who tried to find an English publisher of Berzelius' book <u>Lessons in Animal Chemistry</u> without success. Marcet was a physician at Guy's Hospital and wrote a book on urinary calculi and wrote a book, <u>An Essay on the Chemical History and Medical Treatment of Calculous Disorders.</u> Many of the Animal Chemists analyzed urine calculi since it was a common medical problem and the stone when passed was an accessible object of study. It may be remembered that the Reverent Stephen Halles in the century before, after his ground breaking demonstration of measuring the blood pressure in a horse and the effect on blood pressure of exsanguinations, took to trying to dissolve kidney stones. Marcet tabulated characteristics and test of a variety of calculi such lithic acid, or uric acid stones, "mulberry"or calcium oxalate, triple phosphate, and " bone earth" or calcium phosphate stones. Astley P Cooper, a famous surgeon at Guy's requested Marcet to perform chemical tests on chyle and other fluids on feeding experiments in dogs at the surgeon reported upon. Marcet died about the time Richard Bright began making observations on renal disease at Guy's so he did not participate directly in the circle of Animal Chemists that would contribute to Bright's observation.

Animal Chemist John Bostock

John Bostock, a physician and lecturer in chemistry was one of Richard Bright's original collaborators in studying the urine and blood of the patients with renal disease. The initial 1827 edition of <u>The Case Reports</u> contains three detailed letters from John Bostock to Richard Bright describing his studies of urine and blood from these reported cases. The initial discussion is about the Specific Gravity of the urine under various circumstances. (Specific Gravity is still an item in the urinalysis today, although Homer Smith admonished nephrologists to take their hydrometers to the highest point in the hospital and drop them over, preferring to rely on osmolality.) He reported on high albumin in the urine and low values in blood reporting, " although I am not able to state precisely the amount of the difference." In studying a specimen of "dropsical urine" he reports "We have here, therefore, an example of the blood exhibiting a very great deficiency of albumen, at the same time that we observe the mode in which it passes off from the system by means of the kidney, while this organ has its appropriate office of secreting urea nearly suspended." In the second volume of Cases and Observations, Illustrative of Renal Disease Accompanied with the Secretion of Albuminous Urine, published in the Guy's Hospital Reports in 1838, Bostock reported the presence of urea in hydrocephalic brain fluid in several patients who had seizures as part of their uremic syndrome. Richard Bright gave credit to Doctor Robert Christison of Edinburgh, where Bright as well as several of the other animal chemists had had their medical education, for identifying urea in the blood of several patients with renal disease. The difficulty in performing reliable quantitative chemical analysis for urea as well as other substances was responsible for the clinical – pathological correlations in defining a clinical entity far outdistancing the early feeble attempts at defining the chemical and physiological functions of the kidney. Bright to his credit did not feel that the elevated urea reported in the hydrocephalic fluid of patients with seizures, was a significant etiological factor in this clinical presentation.

Animal Chemist William Prout

William Prout (1785-1850), a physician and Animal Chemist, who received his MD from Edinburgh, as did Bright and many of his circle, was one of the leading Animal Chemists in England. He analyzed a wide variety of plant and animal products and believed that such information would be of value to physicians in diagnosis and treatment of disease. He was most insistent on obtaining purity of both the reagents being used and the product analyzed. His meticulous and laborious purification of urea was described earlier. However his preparation was considered one of the most accurate at the time. Richard Bright in his Gulstonian Lecture 11 On the Functions of the Abdomen and some of the Diagnostic Marks of its Disease, published in London Medical Gazette, vol. X11 1833, remarks "I do not intend to enter into a detailed account of all the indications of disease derived from the urinary secretion- a subject upon which we possess a work from the pen of Dr. Prout, than which one more concise, more accurate, or more philosophic in its character, scarcely exists on any other subject connected with our profession." He was referring to an article in Med-Chir, Trans, 8, 526-549, 1817 on Observations on the Nature of some the Proximate Principles of the Urine. Bright goes on in this Gulstonian Lecture to eschew the methods of the Animal chemists writing,"but still I trust I may be forgiven if, passing over much of this interesting field of inquiry, I enlarge a little upon one favourite topic,-the indications of disease derived from the albuminous condition of the urine", and goes to stress the importance of the finding of albumin with anasarca as a clue to the finding of kidney disease. Prout studied the nature of urinary Calculi, as did many of the Animal Chemists. He discovered that 80% of the content of the urine from a boa constrictor consisted of uric acid. Earlier it had been determined that guano from birds in South America contained uric acid. He also devised a portable hydrometer, probably not unlike the ones used by physicians in much of the twentieth century to measure specific gravity, a measurement that Bright and other Animal Chemists were fond of following . One of Prout's most important discoveries was that hydrochloric acid was present in gastric juice. Previously it had been considered the lactic acid was the agent responsible for the acid in gastric juice. William Beaumont a few years later in studying the French Canadian, Alexis St Martin, who had a gastric fistula created following a gun shot wound of the abdomen, in America confirmed Prout's observation on the presence of gastric acid in the stomach, and in addition recorded the influence of emotions, food, and other factors in its appearance.

Animal Chemist George Owen Rees

George Owen Rees was another of the Animal Chemists –Physicians who obtained early experience in Bright's group at Guy' Hospital studying the newly defined entity renal disease, as characterized by Bright. Unlike many of the other collaborators Rees disliked the postmortem room, turned away because of its pungent ordors, and became a tireless investigator of the chemical study of urine, blood and other organs. He entered Guy's at the age of sixteen as a pupil of Richard Stocker, apothecary to the hospital. He dedicated the second edition of his book, On the Analysis of the Blood and Urine, 1845, "gratitude for the kind encouragement received from you when, as a mere boy, I first entered on the study of pathological chemistry." He was insistent on the need to establish control values in blood and urine for substances to be measured. This continued to be a very hard task, because of the primitive and laborious tasks need in the analysis of various substances. Neither urea nor sugar had been constantly measured in blood of normal subjects. This he was able to do under certain circumstances. In a report in the Guy's Hospital Reports 3, page 398-400, 1838, he isolated sugar in the blood of a diabetic by isolating crystals of sugar after various extractions, involving boiling water, alcohol, and ether, followed by filtration and evaporation to dryness. The ether as considered to remove urea and fatty material .His method was said to reduce the time of analysis from several weeks to several days! He pointed out that tests for albumin in the urine by heat alone might be spurious, urates may be precipitate by HNO_3, phosphates precipitated by heat but dissolved by acid, and bladder stones could produce a positive test for albumin when the kidney was not the diseased organ. Bright in his Gulstonian Lecture 11,not only gave Prout credit as noted above but attributes to Rees the confusion with regard to phosphates mimicking albuminuria, "where urea is unusually abundant, a decomposition takes place by the application of heat, and ammonia is formed, which precipitates the phosphate in a form which it is almost impossible to distinguish by the eye from some albuminous precipitates: such, at least is an explanation of the phenomenon, which has been given me by my friend Mr. Rees, and appears very probable." Bright had great respect for the eye giving true knowledge, as is demonstrated in his meticulous description of the kidney at the autopsy table, and seems to reluctantly agree to a chemical explanation to separated out the similar appearance of precipitates of albumin and phosphate.

A further example of Rees' meticulous and laborious method for the isolation of urea from the blood appears also in the second edition of his Analysis of the Blood and Urine in Health and Disease, 1848:

Examination of Blood supposed to contain Urea

1. Let a portion of serum be accurately weighed and then evaporated to dryness over an open steam-bath.(By using an open steam-bath, we are always certain of keeping the matter of experiment at a heat considerable below 212 degrees Fahrenheit, which is absolutely necessary in these experiments, since urea in dilute solution becomes gradually destroyed if kept at the temperature of boiling water)

2. A quantity of distilled water (amounting to about one ounce for each 200 grains of serum used for experiment) is to be heated to 200 degrees Fahrenheit, and then poured on the dry extract, which must be previously broken up with a sharp spatula. A digestion over the seam-bath for about half and hour is now to be performed; the loss of water by evaporation being supplied occasionally be the experimenter.

3. The digested fluid is to be filtered, and the residue on the filter washed with distilled water (the washings being added to the original liquor.) The whole of the filtered liquor is now to be evaporated to dryness over an open stem-bath, and the residue of the evaporation digested with absolute alcohol, at a gentle heat, for half an hour; care being taken that the loss by evaporation do not materially diminish the bulk of the fluid.

4.   A second filtration is now to be performed, and the filtered fluid must again be evaporated to dryness, and then dissolved in a small portion of lukewarm distilled water. We thus procure an aqueous solution of urea, combined with animal extractive;   to   this   solution   (previously evaporated to the consistence of a thin syrup) we now add a few drops of nitric acid, which causes an effervescence. This mixture must be set aside to crystallize.

5.   Should crystals appear, of the peculiarly characteristic appearance of nitrate of urea, we may conclude the urea is present: indeed, if crystals exist at all after the foregoing process, they must be nitrate of urea; since on principle of the blood that can possibly exist in the last-tested fluid possesses the property of becoming less soluble by the addition of nitric acid.

6.   Crystals being formed in the liquor, we may now proceed to ascertain the proportion of urea. etc. etc.

Prout's description of the isolation of urea from urine had been described. The above description of Rees' method of isolation and quantification of urea from the blood was much more involved and speculative, since urea was not regularly found in normal blood and appeared only with advanced renal failure, as can be seen from Rees' comment " Should crystals appear"

Rees translated from the French, J.J. Berzelius' book, "The Analysis of Inorganic Bodies," and laid much emphasis not only on the purity of reagents, as had Prout, but on simplifying chemical tests so that they could be of use for the clinical practice of medicine. The relationship of Chyle and blood were poorly understood and Rees undertook studies from human material obtained from newly executed criminals. The then current opinion was that chyle was a precursor of blood, but Rees' studies tended to deny this. Rees who tended not to extrapolate from his findings, and pointing out the unknown origin of albumin and urea as products of the liver, hypothesized that the fatty matter of the chyle reacted with nitrogen as well as oxygen in the lung, to produce albumin!.

Rees was involved in medical legal problems and forensic medicine. He denied the presence of Arsenic occurring naturally in bones as had been claimed by the Paris Professor of Medicine and toxicology, M.J.B. Orfila. Rees was involved in a famous case of alleged Strychnine poisoning. This was in the trial of William Palmer accused of poisoning his wife in order to collect on her insurance. Strychnine could not be detected in her body, but it was Rees' testimony that with the chemical tests available Strychnine could not be determined in animals given a lethal dose. The prisoner was convicted on other evidence and the insurance company was saved having to pay out on the deceased insurance policy. In his Lettsomian lectures as published in Lond. Med. Gas. In 1851, he stress that chemical analysis could assist with diagnosis, leading to treatment that might not be possible from other areas of study. (The Numbers today are often the first line of diagnosis, even before examination and other procedures are considered.) But this was the first half of the nineteenth century and Animal Chemistry was in its infancy and had few followers. Rees carried on as a successful medical physician, lecturer, and also a physician at the Pentonville prison, where he advocated hygienic measures, and in 1882 became physician extraordinary to the Queen.

Richard Bright's Recognition of the Animal Chemists

The study of these patients with renal disease was enthusiastically received and two wards were set-aside for Bright to gather together patients with renal disease so that they could be studied in one place rather than scattered throughout the hospital. In effect this represented the first instance of a research project devoted to a single disease entity in a designated area with a director and assistants. There was one male ward of twenty-four beds and a female ward of eighteen beds with a small office and lab set up in between the two wards. Such an ideal set up should have been a harbinger of considerable progress. However, because the original observations of Bright were so cogent and the methods to study further the chemical and physiological aspects of renal disease so primitive that further studies could be predicted to be disappointing. However Bright took up the challenge enthusiastically and with his renal team of Owen Rees, G. Hilaro Barlow, Benjamin Babington and the medical student Mr. Tweedie went to work in earnest. Dr. Barlow later contributed articles on gastrointestinal diseases to the Guy's Hospital Reports and collected many of Bright's papers for publication after his death, and wrote a tribute to Richard Bright in 1861. Bright in his Gulstonian Lecture of 1833, attributes to Barlow and Tweedie studies on the specific gravity of urine in various stages of renal disease. To Benjamin Babington in this same Gulstonian Lecture he gives credit for finding,"no less than fifteen parts in a thousand parts of the serum of the blood to be chiefly urea though somewhat impregnated with other substances." (This would represent 1500mg/DL urea, so that those other "impregnated substances" may have been a factor.) In the Guy's Hospital Report of 1836, under the title of Tabular View of the Morbid Appearances in 100 Cases Connected with Albuminous Urine, he details the clinical and pathological studies that in part were performed with the help of his renal team on the research ward set up for that purpose. Again in the Gulstonian Lecture of 1833, on the <u>Functions of the Abdomen and some of the Diagostic Marks of its Disease,</u> Bright gives credit to the "great assistance from the from the intelligent and zealous co-operation of three of my young friends and pupils, Mr. Barlow, Mr. Tweedie and Mr. Rees. These gentlemen have found, from experiments made upon the urine of two hundred and ninety-six patients, taken at random, in Guy's Hospital, that forty –four, that is, fifteen per cent were coagulated by heat; that thirty-seven, or twelve and half per cent., gave precipitates with nitric acid; and twenty-six, or eight and four fifths per cent., gave precipitates with both." Using this epidemiological approach, and if these "eight and four fifths percent " of patients had underlying renal disease, this would rival the frequency of tuberculosis, probably the most common disease at that time. The subsequent history and progress of the medical student Mr. Tweedie, who was a member of Bright's team, has not been possible to determine.

Vitalism

Throughout the nineteenth century a vital force or Vitalism was widely accepted as an explanation for the complex processes of plants and animals that the burgeoning field of chemistry could not account for. T.C. Litman characterized Vitalism as "the belief in the existence of some operating principle which is not found in organic nature and which distinguishes a living organism from the physico-chemical world." Wohler's demonstration of the production of urea from ammonium cyanate did not eliminate Vitalism in chemical processes. Berzelius and von Liebig had considerable correspondence over the significance of this finding. Beside considering its production as just a rearrangement, Johannes Muller, the German physiologist in the second edition of his <u>Handbuch der physiologie des Menschen</u> suggested that urea was a borderline substance at "the extreme boarder of organic substances and is more of an excrete than a compound with the characteristic properties of organic products." Wohler 's "synthesis" of urea was then either considered a rearrangement or was not germane to the consideration of Vitalism.

Vitalism filled the gaps in the explanation of animal and chemical events that were poorly understood or beyond the capabilities of the emerging nascent chemistry of the early nineteenth. The animal chemists were fond of boiling, evaporating, incinerating, desiccating to explore the nature and composition of materials. How such processes such as the excretion of urine, digestion and locomotion could be carried out in an organism of relatively constant temperature was difficult to imagine. The influence of enzymes, hormonal and other biochemical transformations had not yet been formulated. A hundred years later in 1927 Alfred Cushney's book, "Secretion of the Urine" failed to consider tubular secretion as a possibility in part because it brought up the specter of vitalism, which by that time was not an operative concept.

Prout didn't use the term Vitalism but rather considered " Organic Agents" as an alternative that could vitalize chemical compounds and produce the multitude of reactions responsible for living mater. All the animal chemists, Fourcroy, Von Liebig, Berzelius, Prout, Rees,etc accepted Vitalism. Many considered that more information and advancement of knowledge would make Vitalism less necessary in their thinking. But along with other physical forces such as permeability, weight, gravity, chemical affinities, Vitalism would continue to be considered to explain chemical reactions that involved growth, nutrition and secretion of the urine.

Animal Chemist Henry Bence-Jones

Henry Bence-Jones (1813-1873) is most familiarly known to physicians today in relation to the protein found in the urine in Myeloma, but he was also an important Animal Chemist, just after Richard Bright. Like all the Animal Chemists he was determined to apply methods of chemistry to Medicine and make it more scientific and exact.

H. Bence-Jones after receiving a medical degree, spent two years in Gressen Germany working with Von Liebig, becoming enamored by the latter's theories of oxidative change to explain metabolic processes in the body. Many including Berzelius criticized Von Leibig for the lack of scientific verification of these theories, but Bence-Jones accepted them uncritically. On his return to England, he incorrectly applied the oxidative theory to the production of urea from uric acid with little evidence to support this supposition. He more productively studied the acidity of the urine and presence of phosphate with changes in diet. After a protein meal, acidity increased (pH decreased) and after vegetables the urine acidity decreased (became more alkaline).

In 1845 Bence-Jones examined the urine from a patient with mollities ossium, a type of malignancy of bone, and found that the urine contained a large portion of albumin that had the unusual property of redissolving in boiling nitric acid, a reaction that was unlike albumin that was resistant to being dissolved by heat. This observation was not noticed for a hundred years, F.W.Pittman in 1955 reported that Bence –Jones protein was not albumin but a light chain immunoglobulin.

Bence-Jones worked at St. Georges Hospital rather the Guy's . He began using spectroscopic analysis for trace metals such as lithium. After feeding lithium carbonate to animals found that the lithium diffused into vascular tissues and the humours of the eye very rapidly, remaining in the urine for as much as thirty-nine days. He studied rubidium, strontium as well as thallium and with a fluorescent technique evaluating quinine. He wrote a book On Animal Chemistry, and encouraged the study of chemistry to be taught in the Medical Schools.

Conclusion

All these Animal Chemists in England, Bostek, Babington, Prout, and Rees practiced Medicine, as well as contributing to Animal Chemistry. Richard Bright in two publications in 1827 and 1843 defined the clinical entity bearing his name, Morbus Brightii. This was done with careful clinical description and elegant gross pathology descriptions, correlating these findings with the constant low tech finding of coagulation of the urine. Bright for the most part did not look at the urine otherwise, nor did he have the benefit of microscopic examinations of the pathological material. While he himself could not be considered an Animal Chemist he encouraged those physicians around him to exam the blood, urine and other fluids from his patients with renal failure. They analyzed the urine for its specific gravity, characterized the proteinuria, and made haltingly primitive and laborious studies of the urea content of urine and blood. They used the techniques of the European Chemists, Berzelius, Von Lebig and Fourcroy. As Animal Chemistry would give way to Physiological Chemistry and then to Biochemistry, the function of the kidney and an understanding of renal insufficiency would allow physicians to better understand and care for their patients, the primary aim of the Animal Chemists in the circle of Richard Bright.

Chapter Five

The Therapeutic Spectrum Available to Those Defining a
Newly Recognized Clinical Entity—Bright's Disease

> Sganarelle, It would do you no harm to bleed
> you a little...
>
> Geronte, Why start blood letting when the
> patient's in good health?
>
> Sganarelle, The method is a salutary one. Just as
> one drinks as a precaution against thirst so one
> should be bled in preparation in illnesses to
> come.
>
> Moliere, Le Medicin malgre lui (1673)

Therapeutic options for a disease entity reflect
knowledge of the underlying etiology and pathological
processes, custom and historical precedent, and

available methods of intervention. While tuberculosis was long recognized as a clinical entity and even after its pathological and etiological factors were defined, it was many years before definitive therapeutic measures became effective. In those years of ineffective therapeutic limbo, treatment reflected the available armamentarium and custom of the times; diet, removal to a more conducive climate, sanitariums, exercise after a fever subsidence, and general measures as itemized by Sir William Osler in the first edition of the Principles and Practice of Medicine, 1892. These general measures also included Creosote, Cod-liver Oil, The Hypophosphites and Arsenic. Osler recognized, "No medicinal agents have any special or peculiar action upon tuberculous processes. The influence which they exert is upon the general nutrition, increasing the physiological resistance, and rendering the tissues less susceptible to invasion."

When a new disease entity makes its appearance as with HIV in the 1980s or Bird Flu in 2000, therapeutic measures mirrored the available remedies thought commensurate with and compatible with general theories and understanding of related clinical entities. Similarly when Richard Bright correlated the findings of Dropsy, coagulable urine and small granular kidneys into a clinical entity in his 1827 publication *Reports of Medical Cases Selected with a View of Illustrating the Symptoms and Cure of Diseases by Reference to Morbid Anatomy* his therapeutic options were limited. He was limited by his understanding of the general theories of disease processes of his times and his clinical experience on the effectiveness of such measures available. The passage of time and more critical evaluation of therapeutic options make moot and often engender a modest condescending smirk in the consideration of more ancient attempts to manage disease processes. A recent editorial in the American Journal of Medicine compared the treatment of myocardial infarction in 1945, the date of the original publication of the Journal with current recommendations. State of the art treatment at his earlier date recommended thirty days bed rest, use of Digitalis and debated the use of bed side commodes compared with bathroom privileges. Current Guidelines are just as emphatic on the necessity of antiplatelet agents, beta blockers, ACE inhibitors, interventional procedures and rehabilation measures.

After Richard Bright so brilliantly and succinctly characterized the disease that eventually bore his name, what were his options to manage and hopefully stabilize or possibly cure the underlying disease? We have to recognize that even today with current assumption of alternative etiology of pathogenesis, microscopic and electron microscopy, measurement of blood and urine chemistries, and the use of immunological procedures, definitive therapy of glomerulonephritis remains elusive. Currently inflammation has forced its way back into consideration as an etiological factor in many processes such as arteriosclerosis and heart disease. Inflammation, but in a more ancient context, was the underlying consideration for Richard Bright and those who followed his lead in documenting this new clinical entity of renal disease, Robert Christison and James Crauford Gregory in Scotland, Jonathan Osborne in Ireland and Pierre Rayer in France. Inflammation, having as its root, *inflammo* – to burn, and has its origin in Celsus' *rubor et tumor cum calore et dolore*. Universally in the first half of the nineteenth century inflammation was considered as the underlying process in patients with a sthenic habitus, sanguineous temperment, a full circulation, often with fever and the blood showing a buffy coat. Inflammation was universally considered to be an important factor in this newly described clinical entity of dropsy, coaguable urine and diseased granular, often shrunken kidneys. Its management was a stereotypic response for Depletion therapy. Bleeding, often with the concomitant use of leeches, cathartics, and sweating were the antidote to inflammation and were widely applied. In addition, the use of various herbs and plant products to complement this purpose had had a long and apparently successful history in the management of various diseases. Herman Boerhaave (1668-1738) leading Enlightenment physician from Leiden as well as many of his contemporaries and predecessors, had an herb garden available adjacent to his home to compound and have available medications for daily use. The similarities and differences in the use of therapeutic measures to manage patients with this newly recognized kidney condition will be evaluated comparing Richard Bright's approach with that of his followers, Christison, Gregory, Osbourne and Rayer.

Richard Bright—Reports of Medical Cases Selected with
a View of Illustrating the Symptoms and Cure of
Diseases by a Reference to Morbid Anatomy (1827)

What did Richard Bright recommend for the treatment and management of his newly described clinical entitity? In *Case Reports* Bright indicates, "In the treatment of the disease, as it occurs in sudden attacks of anasarca from intemperance and exposure, in its early stages, and before organic changes have taken place, we have two distinct indications to fulfill; - we have to restore the healthy action of the kidney, and we have to guard continually against those dangerous secondary consequences which may destroy the patient at any period of the disease." Except for the implicit assumption that intemperance and exposure are etiological factors, this introductory statement could have come right out of a current textbook of nephrology. Bright continues, "The two sources of casual danger will be found in inflammatory affections (conditions), more particularly of the serous, sometimes of the mucous membranes, and in the effusion of blood or serum into the brain and the consequent occurrence of apoplexy." There we have it, *inflammatory affections,* as well as his concern with the neurological complication in the cases he described. Bright continues, " Hence it is that in the earl stages of the disease it will generally be indispensably necessary to have recourse to active depletion." Bright specifies his treatment further, "In a great many instances the abstraction of blood generally has been productive of speedy good effects; and in other cases it has seemed to me, that by drawing blood locally by cupping from the loins much good has been effected.

Bleeding had been practiced in moderation in Ancient times, but became a more florid therapeutic depletion measure in the first part of the nineteenth century. Cupping is an ancient procedure form Chinese practice in which a cup, the rim often heated, is applied to the skin as a suction device so that the skin and superficial skin and muscle layers are drawn into and held in the cup. Wet cupping implies making an incision into the skin so that blood and serum can be drawn up into the cup. Modern acupunturist employ cupping for a wide variety of conditions. The Jews of Russia and Eastern Europe frequently used cupping and there is a Yiddish expression describing the therapeutic options for a terminally ill patient, " Es vet helfen wie ain toten bankas—It will help like giving a dead person Bankas (Russian for cups).

Bright next takes up Purgatives as a form of depletion therapy. "Purgatives generally act well." Elaterium is his first choice. The common name for Elaterium is *Squirting cucumber.* It is a an energetic hydragogue laxative, producing copious watery stools with even low dosage of ¼ grain" He cites the patient Evans, case XIV in which Elaterium "evidently gave much relief" Evans was "a Welchman of remarkably stout frame presenting with "general anasarca to a great extent." Extract,

Elaterii prescribed and he reports "the swelling rather diminishes." Bright continues commenting on the effectivness of Elaterium, "The pills have purged him very often, with much pain before they act, and much sickness, urine rather increased. Swelling a good deal reduced; urine in sixteen hours six pints and a half." Continuing on the subject of purgatives, Bright states, " all the saline laxatives which unite a certain degree of diuretic power are decidedly useful. Amongst these I have found the Supertartrate of Potash the most efficacious." Supertartrate of Potash or potassium bitartrate is commonly called Cream of Tartar, the acidic potassium salt of tartaric acid, $KC_4H_5O_6$ is today used as a leavening agent in baking powders. It is to be distinguished from sodium potassium tartrate or Rochelle salt. Bright goes on to discuss the preferred method of using such agents, " the best mode of exhibiting it when the stomach will admit, is by directing the patient to take a large draught of a mixture containing more of the salt (supertartrate of potash) than the water will dissolve, the first thing in the morning: and it will be seen that in some cases I have almost trusted entirely to this remedy. Where the stomach will not bear this mode of administering purgative, the combination of Jalap, Supertartrate of Potash and a little Ginger repeated from time to time answers well, or even frequent doses of Castor Oil have been very useful." Jalop is a tuberous root of *Exogonuim purga*, Jalapa is a city in Mexico. Castor Oil is a laxative familiar to everyone. It is made from the seeds of the Castor Oil plant, *Ricinus communis,* anative plant from India. It contains Palmitic and several other fatty acids but Ricinoleic acid which is though to be the active agent responsible for its purgative action. It was known to Herodotus in the fourth century B.C. as an agent much used by the Egyptians and in whose tombs are found are found the *Ricinus* seeds. Ginger also known by everyone and is a plant originally from Southern China and cultivated in subtropic Asia especially India. The name is from the Greek *singiberis*. It is used to flavor foods and by Bright to take the edge off the Jalap/Supertartrate of Potash mixture. Ginger ale a popular soft drink in America but does not contain ginger, rather is a plant extract with carbonated water and sugar. Richard Bright prescribed the combination of Jalap and Potassium Supertartrate of Case XVlll, William Brooks presenting with generalized edema whose urine coagulates by heat, and whose bowels were "confined." Rx: *Habeat Pulveris Jalap. Cum Potass. Supertartrate.* He also prescribed *Ol. Ricini* or Castor oil, referring to Ricinoleic acid, the active principal.

Bright next takes up Diuretics and as they were derived at that time from herbal medicine the term had a broader meaning that just to facilitate an increase in urine flow as is our understanding today. Rather the action of a diuretic could refer to any effect on the urinary system, not only to increase flow of urine but to act as a soothing effect or demulcent on the urinary bladder or urethra. So that Bright's listing of agents such as narcotics and anticholinergic compounds are to be considered in the broader definition of diuretics in the more traditional herbal connotation. With this in mind, it will be more understandable that Bright should states that," The diuretic remedy which I have generally used was been the Squill in its different forms: but it has always acted best when given in combination with Hyoscyamus, or when a grain of Opium has been prescribed. Squill is from the bulb of a plant, *Urginea scilla* containing a glucoside of uncertain composition. In ancient times it was used for cough and in the mediaeval period for its alleged diuretic action. Hyoscyamus or Henbane is related to Belladonna/atropine. Henbane is an European herb, all parts of the plant are of some medicinal value, but it is the leaves and seeds that are more useful. Hyoscyamus is a narcotic similar to stramonium and belladonna producing the well known dryness of mouth, papillary dilatation, and tachycardia and mental changes with larger doses. It has some affect on bladder and urethra to relieve spasm and irritation. The consideration of Hysocyamus and Opium as diuretics probably relate to these effects, since in the very next sentence Bright states, "Indeed I cannot but consider this (the combination of Hyocyamus and Opium) an important part of the treatment, with a view to diminish the *irritation* of the kidneys, as well as to allay the general disturbance which must necessarily result to the constitution, from the circulation of blood which has been so imperfectly acted upon by these organs." Opium, of course is of ancient linage having been cultivated in Mesopotamia over five thousand years ago. It is probably the most well known and useful of currently used drugs that made up Richard Bright's armamentarium. It is doubtful if it contributed to the diuretic potency in combination with Squill, which like Digitalis may have been helpful if there was cardiac involvement. What would Richard Bright think of the efficacy of modern diuretics?

Continuing under the heading of Diuretic Remedy, Bright next takes up Digitalis, a drug like opium very familiar to physicians today, since its description by William Withering in 1785, *Account of Foxglove and Some of Its Medical Uses.* Returning to Bright, "Digitalis has in some instances been cautiously administered with temporary advantage, and seems by its power of checking the circulation to be well adapted to those cases where the pulse is sharp, as frequently occurs throughout the whole progress of this disease." Withering recommended Foxglove for dropsy, irrespective of its cause, being cautious about the dose and prevention of toxicity. Bright's contribution was to define a subset of those patients with dropsy that had renal disease alone and in the above statement seems to recognize the benefits of Digitalis to "check the circulation ....where the pulse is sharp." In the case of Plume, Digitalis acted well: in the treatment of Thomas it entirely failed." Eliza Plum was a single woman, age 18, affected with anasarca, pulse sharp. Digitalis was added to a mixture of Scille and Hydrarg. Oxyd. (Squill and Mercury oxide, see below for a discussion of mercury)) " with the addition of ten drops of tincture of digitalis to each dose of the mixture and half a grain of opium at bed-time." After "once or twice moderate bleedings were had recourse to when the pulse was sharp", and after Antimonii tartarizat. (ammonium tartrate), Jalap, Balsam. Peruvian Linimentum (Peruvian Balsam - see below), cupping, Scillae and Hyoscyam. (Hyoscymus), "edema gone from the eyelids, feels better, and continues to pass a tolerably natural quantity of urine." Plum was still under observation at time of publication of *Case Reports*. Such was a case where Digitalis apparently, along with a plethora of other agents, "acted well." In the case of Hugh Thomas, a stout looking sailor of 34 years presenting "the most decided oedema of the lower legs, urine scanty", after gray oxide of mercury with squills, tartrate of potash "with a little of the tincture of digitalis ...he improved for some days, his urine rather increased." However this was only temporary and "it was necessary to give purgatives, Jalap and Supertartrate of Potash (Cream of Tartar) ... the urine becoming scanty and he died on the 14th." Digitalis along with several other drugs, was considered by Bright to have "entirely failed."

Continuing further with Bright's recommendation for a Diuretic Remedy, Under certain circumstances, more particularly when the more inflammatory stage of the disease has subsided, Turpentine employed in the mode of friction (rubbing), and the Peruvian balsam administered internally, have seemed decidedly useful. Turpentine is a yellow to brown semifluid oleoresin exuded from the sapwood of pines, firs, and other conifers. It contains an essential oil and a type of resin called rosin. While used today as a solvent and drying agent in paints, it was commonly used as an irritating counter irritant. South American balsam trees, especially that from Peru, today is used in cough mixtures and in the vapour when inhaled for catarrh. As noted above Elisa Polum was treated with Peruvian Balsam.

Richard Bright next takes up the "most important questions in the treatment of this class of dropsies, the propriety of employing Mercury. It is consistent with the most successful treatment of many forms of inflammatory disease, that we should have recourse to the valuable combination of Calomel with Opium" Mercury was know to the physicians of antiquity but not used as a medication, being considered more as a poison, like our current consideration of Mercury in fish or from environmental waste. Avicenna was among the first of the Arabian physicians to use it orally as well as externally. Paraselsus like wise recommended it as a medication. Calomel (Gr. *kalos*—fair or beautiful plus *melas* black) is mercuous chloride used as treatment for syphilis and widely considered as a treatment of inflammatory conditions in the 18th century and a favorite of Benjamin Rush in America. In considering mercury however, Bright becomes very insightful, "still however, the cases which have proved most successful in my own practice, have generally been those in which I have rigidly abstained from the use of mercury." As we can see from the description of therapeutic measures noted previously, he was not entirely opposed to the use of mercury, however he was astute to recognize that toxicity from mercury, ptyalism, in these group of patient. He indicates that while "the free use of mercury to complete ptyalism has not prevented the patients from deriving great, perhaps perfect relief, from the remedies with which it was combined, these remedies having been bleeding, purging and diuretics. ...there is one circumstance which most materially limits our power of employing it, and that is the violent and rapidity with which the ptyalism often comes on, (resulting in) the gums and cheeks not being capable of supporting the process of ulceration and often passing into a state of gangrene" Bright seems to have stumbled upon the fact that mercury toxicity is more easily produced in renal insufficiency.

In the concluding paragraphs on treatment, Bright become cautious about any treatment, especially when the "morbid deposit in the kidney becomes preternaturally hard (irreversible), we can only employ palliative remedies. If we could ascertain by well marked symptoms the existence of this state, probably the great advantage we should gain from the knowledge, would he in its restraining us from adopting those more active remedies which would be apt to wear out the powers of life, without affording any permanent relief to the organs affected." Sir William Osler probably read these words to support his dictum of therapeutic conservatism.

In a concluding paragraph on treatment, Richard Bight indicates that,"occasionally we find anasarca even with coagulable urine so marked by debility that tonics give decided relief; probably it is as a tonic that the Uva Ursi is sometimes useful." The common name for Uva Ursi is Bearberry, botanical name Arctostaphylos, from the Latin meaning bear grape. It is a small shrub widely distributed and related to the Arbutus. The plant may have been given this name from the notion that bears eat the fruit or from its disagreeable flavor which only bears would like. The dried leaves are used medicinally. It is said to have a soothing and astringent effect with marked diuretic action and of value in diseases of the bladder and kidneys as well as having a diuretic action, considered due to the action of the glucoside Arbutin.

In addition to these therapeutic measures outlined by Dr. Bright in the section labeled Observations on the Treatment in his *Case Reports* of 1827, Bright used many other procedures and treatments, all prescriptions written in Latin.

These include Dover's powder, a combination of opium and ipecac plus other agents – salt peter (KNO3), Tartar vitriolated KSO4), and liquorish) was first described by the British physician, Thomas Dover, (1660-1742) originally in 1732 advocated for relief of gout. Later is was considered to combine the pain relieving action of opium and the diaphoretic action of the combination of opium and ipecac. Ipecac is a plant from Brazil and the name is from the Portuguese from of the native word, i-*pe-kaa-guene,* meaning road-sick making plant, the action occasional used today to induce vomiting, present in the root of Ipecacuanga as Emetine. Bright's first patient, John King, a sailor, "accustomed to take considerable quantities of spirits", presenting with pain in the loins and anasarca, received   *Hydrarg. Oxydi cinerei, Pilul. Scillae compos.* and *Opii purificat* (Mercuric oxide, Squill, and Opium. He also received a combination of *Vini Ipecacuanhae, Olei Ricini, cum Tinct. Opii* (Ipecac wine, castor oil and opium). John King also received *Mittatur sanguis ad f. oz x* (a phlebotomy of 300 ml of blood) and *Applicetur Empl. Cantharidis Sterno.* (application of a poultice of Cantharidis to the sternum). Canthardes or Spanish fly / blisterbeetle is an insect the wings of which contain an intense irritating substance which the beetle uses as a defensive mechanism, and used therapeutical as and a blistering agent. (The supposed action of increasing male sexuality is related to it strongly irritating the genito-urinary tract, sexual activity being used to relieve the intense discomfort) Leonard Evans,

Case XIV "a Welshman of remarkably stout frame, said to have been the strongest man out of 1400 in Deptford dock yard" presenting with anasarca received *Extract. Elaterii* (mentioned as a purgative in Bright's Observation on Treatment), as well as *Spartii scoparii* (Broom or Broom tops, *Spartium scoparium*, a common shrub indigenous to England, used in ancient Anglo-Saxon medicine, and as a heraldic symbol. *Sparteine* is considered the active principal along with *Scoparin* responsible for its action a weak diuretic and cathartic.)

Still another patient from Bright's reports that gives a sampling of his therapeutic options was Thomas Drudget age 37, Case XIII "was a carman, in the habit of drinking a little, while in his work, but by no means an intemperate man, coming home very regularly and always passing his evening with his family." He presented with nausea, oedema with "legs so swollen that he could not button the knees of his small-clothes." His first treatment was *Appicentur Cucurbitulae cruente Scrob.Cordis* (wet cupping over the heart) While cupping goes back to China, the Romans used a gourd, the hard rind of a fruit of the member of the family Cucurbitaceae. The Latin name used in medicine for cupping was "Cucurbitula", and this was its designation exclusively used by Bright as an indication for cupping. Cupping originated in China. Horns of animals were used early and those used by the Romans often were made of brass. Glass cups are most popular later. They would be heated and the vacuum provided by the removal of oxygen would act as a suction device as it is placed on the skin. Wet cupping implied the placing of an incision and the suction cups applied over the incision to remove a relatively small amount of blood. Dry cupping was performed without on incision or removing any blood was widely used until just recently and has had a resurgence of popularity in alternative medicine.

Additional therapeutic items as carefully laid out in
Latin by Richard Bright as part of the treatment for those
patients described in the 1827 *Case Reports* include
Extr.Conii, or Conium (water hemlock), an antcholinergic
agent in the family with Pilocarpine, probably used for
its effect in increasing secretions and sweating. John
King, Bright's first patient received this as well as a
mixture of *Camphorae,* or Camphor from wood
distillation, probably considered a stimulant, since the
patient was becoming more depressed." This was mixed
with *Liquor. Ammoniae Acetat,* ammonium acetate,
similar to Spirits of Mindereri, described by Dr.
Raymund Minderer of Augsburg in 1619 as a cathartic
and diuretic, and *Spir. Aether. Nitr,* volatile spirt of nitric
acid. This same John King also received a mixture of
Antimonii tartarizate, Antimony tartrate, *Opii purificati,*
purified opium and *Theriacae q.s.,* an ancient
polypharmacutical produce of sixty four ingredients
mixed with honey and said to be effective against
poisons. As a flavoring agent *Zingib. Radicis,* root of the
ginger plant, Latin *Zingiber,* was frequently added to
the combination of Elatarium and Cream of tarter. *Pulv.
Rhei,* pulverized Radix Rhei, or Chinese rhubarb was
likewise added to mercury preparation, probably to
augment the laxative affect, as suggested by the
comment "bowels not well opened' as reported in Case
XV William Roederik who was reported to be
improving, "approaching a state of convalescence; but
unfortunately, without any obvious cause, his disease
took a less favorable turn." He remained under Dr.
Bright's care with " all the symptoms of confirmed
disorganization of the kidneys at the time of publication
of the *Case Reports.* This listing does not exhaust the
therapeutic options available to Richard Bright but
gives a flavor to the variety of his choices.

While bleeding and cupping depletion therapy of all
varieties, tonics, etc were frequently employed by

Richard Bright, there is no record in the *Case Reports* of the use of leeches. Leeches were very vigorously and commonly used among the physicians who preceeded and followed in Bright's steps to further characterize and give meaning to the triad of dropsy, coagulable urine and kidney pathology, such as Robert Christison, Pierre Rayer and others to be evaluated for their therapeutic options. This was the era of the explosive use of leeches to augment in a more selective way blood loss as part of the general depletion measures. Richard Bright's eschewing this popular therapy has no obvious explanation.

A possible clue to this lack of utilization of leeches by Dr. Bright at Guy's Hospital may come from *An Address* delivered by Dr. Charles J. Hare at the Annual Meeting of the Metropolitan Counties Branch as published in the *British Medical Journal* in July 28, 1883. He reviews how drugs and treatment pass in and out of fashion at the London Hospital during the years1832 through 1882. Hospitals such as Bartholmew's and St George's are reported to have used 97,000 and 21,000 leeches respectively in the ten year period ending 1832, however Guy's Hospital and several others indicate no use of leeches during this time. While these results may reflect difficulty in obtaining accurate information, it is possible that Bright's eschewing the use of leeches which were so popular at other hospitals, Scotland and Paris, may have been out of fashion at Guy's Hospital.

Influence of Medical School Training on the Therapeutic Choices Available to Richard Bright and Robert Christison

Robert Christison of Edinburgh Scottland, along with Bright and Pierre Rayer of Paris, represent the dominant pioneers in the establishment of the clinical recognition of kidney disease. Bright and Christison both attended medical school at Edinburgh, Bright graduating in 1813 and Christison in 1819. William Cullen had been a major force at Edinburgh in the last part of the eighteenth century and both came under the influence of similar mentors advocating a therapeutic spectrum emphasizing inflammation as an underlying theoretical principle and depletion as its antedote .According to John Thompson in his *An Account of the Life, Lectures, and Writings of William Cullen,* " There can be little doubt that it is to trials made by him (William Cullen) in the clinical wards of the Royal Infirmary that we owe, in a considerable degree, the introduction into general practice in this country of various powerful articles of the material medica which are now in daily use, such as Cream of Tartar, Hyosciamus, Cicuta (Water Hemlock, *Cicutoxin*, from Ciuta virosa, a CNS medullary stimulant like Picrotosin), James Powder, (Antimony/calcium phosphate) or Pulvis Antimonialis and Tartar Emetic, the last of which he was accustomed to employ in all febrile affections accompanied with inflammatory action ..." All of these preparations are familiar from the armementarium of Richard Bright and will be shown being used similarly by Robert Chrisitison. In addition J. Worth Estes in his *Dictionary of Protopharmacology,* designates William Cullen as advocating "blood letting as one of the most powerful means of dimininshing the activity of the whole body especially of the sanguiferous (circulatory) system, and it must therefore be the most effectual means of moderating the violence of reaction in fever." The choice of therapeutic agents as well as the basis for blood letting had the authority of William Cullen for students such as Bright and Christison.

Prominent at Edinburgh following Cullen was Dr. James Gregory, famous for his purging powders, described by Christison in his autobiography as. "Gregorian Physic – free blood letting, the cold affusion (pouring water on the part of the body for reducing fever), brisk purging, frequent blisters and the nauseating action of tartar emetic – came to rule medical practice for many year, in all quarters throughout the British Islands and the Colonies" In view of their similar training and environment it can be anticipated that Christian and Bright would share a similar spectrum of therapeutic measures. The Edinburgh School trained their students in the examination of the patient and attention to anatomical findings at autopsy. Physiological and chemical considerations were in their infancy. On the other hand, bland unquestioning acceptance of the value and appropriateness of a theory of disease processes and therapeutic principles were counter to the emphasis on clinical observation with autopsy confirmation at death. Such clinical findings with autopsy and gross pathological correlations were to allow recognition of new clinical entities such as Bright's Disease, Addison's Disease and others. It was not in the air to challenge the basic assumption of disease processes and organ based etiology of disease was in its infancy, stifling a more rational basis for therapeutics. The tools that the Edinburgh school provided were uniquely suited to dissecting out the correlations that made possible a recognition of the kidney as the focus of attention where dropsy and coaguable urine intersected, but the therapeutic implications of this correlation were blinded by ancient, outmoded, and unproven theories. Therefore it is not unexpected that Christison and Bright would share many of the basic underlying principles of the pathogenesis of disease, inflammation being of prime concern and depletion therapy being the accepted therapeutic maneuver to counter it. A through going revision of therapeutic principles would take French and German physiological and chemical insights into the basic concepts of disease and place therapeutic considerations on a firmer foundation.

Robert Christison's of Edinburgh Contributions to the Therapeutic Spectrum of Richard Bright's Newly Described Disease Entity

Sir Robert Christison of the Royal Infirmary in Edinburgh was the first to confirm and champion the observation of Richard Bright. The first report of 1829 *Observation on the Variety of Dropsy which Depends on Kidney Disease* was two years after Bright's initial *Case Reports* of 1827. He enthusiastically confirmed his findings and reported seven cases of his own. The dependency of some cases of Dropsy on a peculiar organic disease of the kidney was lately pointed out by Richard Bright of Guy's Hospital. <u>Since that time I am not aware that any other physician has publicaly noticed this discovery or endeavored to confirm or extend the statement of Dr. Bright."</u>

In his second publication of 1839 he added an additional 39 cases and reported important chemical analyses of the blood and urine, confirming the presence of urea in elevated amounts, by devious and crude chemical procedures, but putting some physiological and chemical parameters on the disease process. Were his therapeutic measures any more advanced or counter to those detailed by Bright? Except for the vigorous use of leeches, Christison's methods of treatment of this newly recognized disease entity were essentially a mirror image, with minor variations from the Edinburgh school of therapeutics, bleeding, cupping, laxatives, merurials, etc.

As an example the therapeutic measures employed in Robert Irving, Case 1, 58 years old, a robust of short stature who presented with edemal of legs and an enlarged abdomen. "He was unable to ascribe any cause to this except general exposure to viscissitudes of temperature. He had a battered dissipated appearance and allowed he had had an interperate life. (Both Christison and Bright considered exposure to cold and alcohol prime etiological factors in the cause of the condition.) His urine produced a copius flocculent precipitate when heated." His treatment consisted of:

> Squill pills, a little Mercury and Digitalis Since the Mercury affected his mouth, (ulceration) it was discontinued. Dysentery was treated with Opium. Supertartrate of Potassium given, 12 ounces of blood drawn from a vein. Because of symptoms of a cough and shortness of breath— a large blister was applied to the sternum

Having been admitted on 7/28/1828 the patient gradually improved and was dismissed on 11/2/1828 (his admission of almost 4 months was not challenged by the insurance agencies!) However he was readmitted two and one half months latter with similar symptoms and was treated with laxatives, mercurials and Digitalis and succumbed to his disease, autopsy confirming granular kidneys.

While the treatment of Robert Irving was very similar to that documented by Richard Bright, a second patient Robert Walker, 32 years old was treated not only with laxative, wine (infrequently noted by Bright), morphine and blisters over the head for mental changes, but twice received twenty leeches first to the loins (to influence the kidneys) and then to the head as seizures occurred. One half of the first ten patients reported in the 1839 edition of *Granular Degeneration* employed leeches. Leeches had been occasionally used since antiquity but it was not until Francois Joseph Victor Broussais, a surgeon in Napolean's Grand Armee advocated their use in the second decade of the nineteenth century as an alternative to blood letting or wet cupping in the treatment of inflammation, being able to be applied in localized areas. The use of leeches spread throughout Europe and England and even to America where Benjamin Rush became an enthusiastic proponent.

Treatment of the Primary Disease

Christison's principals of treatment are summarized in his 1839 book on *Granular Degeneration*. For treatment of the primary disease he suggested a "rigorous antiphologistic remedy of blood letting used best in the early stage unless contraindicated by age or constitutional infirmity. Christison continues, " other depletion measures such as leeches and cupping to the loins, especially serviceable for flank pain are to be used. The antiphlogistic regimen should in no case be relaxed till forces of the circulation are broken. The body should always be warmly clothed, intelligently protected against sudden exposure to cold, especially cold and wet together with a general flannel dress which should be worn constantly" (This attention to the use of flannels to prevent chilling had its echoes as late as the 1892 edition of Sir William Osler's *Principals and Practice of Medicine.)*

Christison recommended counterirritants as additional depletion measures and considered blisters, Setons and Issues. Bright did not seem to employ setons and issues. In this procedure a strip of silk or linen is drawn through a wound in the skin to facilitate the release of serum or pus, much as blisters were raised with Cantharis, thus making a tract or fistula.

What did Christison mean by a "vigorous antiphologistic remedy"? An antiphlogistic medicine was used to neutralize fevers. *Phlogiston* is from the Greek for fire and was considered to be present in combustible substances. Robert Boyle in 1669 had shown the importance of air for both combustion and life. Georg Ernst Stahl in Vienna had postulated a substance he called Phlogiston given off when a candle burns, which no longer supported combustion. Joseph Priestly in England who was later to come to America, an early discoverer of what would later be labeled oxygen, indicated that phlogisticated air can be restored by green plants. Physicians reasoned that a febrile patient with a tachycardia, and other signs of inflammation were to be likened to Phlogiston and devised agents, such as bleeding and other measures to counteract it. Joseph Black of Scotland and later Lavoisier the discoverer of oxygen performed experiments that doubted the existence of Phlogiston, but the medical profession clung to the antiphlogistic theory to treat inflammation. William Cullen as previously noted was instrumental in promulgating bleeding, blisters, and other depletion measures as antiphlogistic measures.

Diaphoretic measures for the induction of sweating are next considered by Christison to provide "vigorous antiphlogistic remedies" as a method of cutaneous transpiration for the primary disease. He considered Dover Powder (Ipecac and Opium) a favorite of Richard Bright. While in large doses the Ipecac is an emetic and is occasionally used today for this purpose, in smaller doses it is a diaphoretic action. In addition, the Acetate of Ammonia or Spirits of Mindererus, a preparation introduced by Dr. Raymond Minderer in Augsberg in 1610 as well as Extract of Hyoscyamus and James Powder were considered as diaphoretic measures. Hyoscyamus nigra was obtained from the leaves, root and seeds of black Henbane, similar to opium without its constipating action. It is recognized today as a potent narcotic with actions like stramonium and Belladonna with dryness of the mouth, flushing of the face and neurological effects and I would judge very little in the way of diaphoresis. It had been introduced by Dr. Gente Storch in Vienna in 1762. Warm baths were used as well and promolgated by Dr Jonathan Osborne, recognized as Ireland's first Nephrologist. His *On the Nature and Treatment of Dropscial Diseases* touted "suppressed perspiration" as the major factor in the development of dropsy. In addition to warm baths Osborne recommended steam baths including immersion of an extremity in a vapour bath. Christison states, "no one can question the propriety of the diaphoreic method in the primary disease, citing Bright on its superiority over diuretics. While Osborne boasted that, " I have never seen it fail to produce favorable results", Christison considered this statement as over optimistic. (It will be recalled that Moliere in his *Le Malade imaginaire* gave the name of Mr. Diafiorus (diaphoresis) to one of his doctors. The other of coarse he labeled Mr. Purgon)

Laxatives were likewise an important part of the depletion regime and Christison recommended Colocynth mass for this purpose. Colocynth is from the dried pulp of the unripe but full grown fruit of *Citrullus colocynthus* from the pulp of fruit of *Citrullus colcynthus* a vigorous and potent cathartic, inhibiting the small bowel inhibiting the reabsorption of water. Other purgatives included those commonly used by Bright and others at this period included Gambage, " the purgative I have most frequently employed." The rough looking gambage of Ceylon was preferred over the variety from Siam. Elaterium and Bitartrate of Potash (Potassium, Sodium Tartrate or Cream of Tartar) were also employed.

Diuretics were next considered. While mercury was not only a diuretic but; had a reputation for its effect as an antiphlogistic remedy in general by "subduing inflammation and removing glandular obstruction", Christison follows Bright's advice "that it is of no use or service in the primary disease." While Bright employed mercury frequently, especially in combination with squill and digitalis, was more cautious in his 1836 publication, *Cases and Observations, Illustrative of Renal Disease Accompainied with the Secretion of Albuinous Urine,* Published in Volume 1 of the Guy's Hospital Reports. He refers to Dr. Barlow of Bath, Dr. Blackall, and Dr. Osborne of Dublin all of whom had reported on adverse side effects with minimal benefits. Bright continues, "When I first published upon this subject, I stated that I had seen much decided mischief from the use of this remedy; yet that I had undoubtedly seen well-marked cases, in which the free use of mercury, even to complete ptyalism, have at leasst not prevented the patients from deriving great, perhaps even perfect relief from the remedies with which it was combined...yet I am bound to say that these cases are rare while the instances of failure and obvious injury from this remedy are numerous." (six of the first ten cases reported by Bright in the original 1827 *Case Reports* where given mercury and several cases on repeated occasions.) Christisian followed this revised view of Bright in treating fluid retention in the primary disease.

Treatment of the Secondary Affection

Christison considered these secondary affection, 1) anasarca, 2) gastrointestinal changes including diarrhea and vomiting and 3) neurological changes such as coma and generalized irritability as " the principal source of danger, the chief cause of discomfort and if they can be successfully warded off or removed the primary disease will give rise to little uneasiness." In addition to the Digitalis, Cream of Tartar with mercury pill as noted above, the list of agents included: 1) Hydragogue cathartics such as Gamboge, 2) Squill, 3) Infusion of Broom Tops, 3) Spirit of Nitric ether, 4) Hollands with water. Broom tops comes from a plant widely grown in Europe having long tough slender branches closely bunched together suitable for broom making that has as its pharmacogical   agent *Sparteine* and *Scoparine,* glucosides that have weak diuretics and cathartic properties. Hollands with water I could not find in standard pharmacological text of the day, but rather in the 3 rd International Websters Dictionary is listed as a gin made in Holland, and could be considered as a gin and tonic of its day.

Purgatives were considered by Christison as a method of removing ascetic fluid and effusions, and "is now less in vogue than formally, but the prejudice against purgatives is carried out by many a great deal too far." Christison recommended Gambage, a powerful laxative, to be used sparingly as an agent to remove ascitic fluid, but Elaterium and Cream of Tartar (Bitartrate of Potash or K Na Tartrate) more frequently. Direct puncture of skin which he refers to as acupuncture (Southey didn't perfect his tube until several decades later) was sometimes used but the tendency to "erythema or gangrene was recognized.

For GI manifestations, opium and astringents such as Lead acetate were considered for diarrhea. *Cerussa acetate or* lead acetate was used as a styptic astringent (both a binding or contracting agent), as an anti-diaphoretic or and anti-inflammatory sedative. A blister to the abdomen for nausea and vomiting was advocated. Blisters were commonly produced by application of a blistering agent such as Cantharis or Spanish fly to remove fluid into the blister or act as a counter irritant. For "ordinary dyspepsia", Christison considered Bitters (a bitter-tasting tonic drug that stumulates the appetite- i.e., an appetizer, by virtue of its local irritant action in the stomach) These included "antacids and other familiar remedies" These familiar remedies included Brandy and for antiacids, ten grs. Magnesia and bicarbonate of soda (a familiar remedy for us today) and Soda of Potash (potassium bicarbonate —potential harm of potassium containing drugs was not recognized at that time.) Also recommended was a stimulant draught of ether, which could be defined as a volatile spirited drink. Hydrochloric acid, one or two drops "before meals sometimes enables the stomach to retain and digest. Opium was used for vomiting from irritability." And finally to control the gastrointestinal symptoms associated with Granular Degeneration, Christisin recommends Creasotum. Creosote is a volital oil first obtained by the destuctive distillaion of wood by Berman natural philosopher Baron Karl von Reichenbach in 1827. How it would affect the GI tract favorably is uncertain but if the dates of its introduction into medicine are correct, it would have been a relatively recent additon to pharmacological agents, since Christison's book, *On Granular Degeneration* was published in 1839. Christison recognized the ubiquitous presence and intractability of gastro intestinal symptoms in renal failure as can be seen by the following quotation: "The physician however although he may be disappointed ought to experience no surprise on finding that all of the above mentioned measures prove ineffective for dyspepsia and chronic vomiting are almost always troublesome when associated with granular kidneys and in some, cause for the most prominent affection and will not yield to any treatment."

For coma or other neurological signs, a brisk purgation, diuretics, or more often leaches to the temple was suggested. Calomel was likewise considered. Blood letting was considered indicated and the"effect of free evacuation of blood was of unquestionable benefit." Christisian and all of his colleagues recognized the dire consequences or coma and similar neurological events.

Christison unlike Bright's original publication of 1827, recognized the possibility of stabilization of the condition and even cure. Active, vigorous antiphlogistic considered in the primary disease and even that discussed in the secondary affections were considered unwarranted. Christison writes as follows:

> When granular disorganization of the kidney has attained the middle or advanced stage or when it puts on the chronic form containment there is little room for active treatment. The Physician can scarsely exercise hope to eradicate it. Still observation has satisfactorily proved that in this condition much may be done for improving health and prolonging life. There is need to arrest the progress of the disorganization as well as to remove and prevent secondary disorders.

To that end Christison recommends the following: "Diet, avoid unusual irritation of the kidneys, maintaince of cutaneous transpiration by warm clothing and occasional warm baths, enforcement of regular active exercising, moderation of food and drink, selection of both nutritious and easily digestible foods, preponderance of vegetable food, abstinence from spirituous liquors as well as sparing use of wine." William Osler must have considered this advice in promulgating his conservative brand of therapeutics.

In summary let us look at a typical case that presented for Robert Christison's care and treatment, #29 James Mossman, a 42 year old harbour porter. He was described as tall, slender robust, and addicted to intemperance. (the implication of alcohol as well as exposure to cold or wet in most other cases was considered a universal etiological factor) He was attacked the middle of February 1836 win a violent inflammation of the lungs, indicated by a very hurried cough, short of breath, with viscus frothy rusty sputum and dullness to percussion at the left lung base. The diagnosis of a severe case of pneumonia was made (even in the absence of auscultation, chest X-ray or CT scan). These findings demanded treatment of acute inflammatory symptoms including:

Immediately the withdrawing of a large quantity of blood.

Nauseating doses of tartar emetic

Calomel/opium

Leeches applied repeatedly to the side of the chest in great number.

By the end of February (about six weeks) the patient was fairly convalescent. He still had left sided pulmonary signs. By the middle of March urine which was initially not coaguable, was reduced in volume volume and coagulated with heat. Mr. Mossman had considerable edema and became drowsy. The diagnosis of Granular Disorganization of the kidneys was now established. Medications included Digitalis, Squill, Bitartrate of Potash. The pulse slowed to 52/min. as Digitalis acted on the heart. Addition of mercury seemed to improve the edema.

Blood drawn at the appearance of the anasarca was subjected to Christison's unique primitive chemical technique, described in a footnote earlier in the discussion. A small portion of the serum was evaporated to dryness, boiled with alcohol, treated with Nitric acid resulting in a "distinct though not abundant crystallization of brownish pearly scales", which was considered urea. Hematosin (Hgb) was low 755 parts/10,000 of blood. (Christison had previously determined in two "healthy" middle aged males that 1535 parts was normal, so that Mossman had a Hemoglobin of about 7.5 gm/dl.

By the end of March the edema and drowsiness had disappeared. Therapy was abandoned with the patient gaining strength, although left sided pulmonary signs remained. By the end of June (five and one half months) he could walk eight miles. The urine was cherry red and was moderately coagulable. In the June of the subsequent year, Dr. Christison chanced to meet Mr. Mossman at work as a porter!

There follows a discussion as to the influence of the mercurial action on improving the patient. The success here experienced under a diuretic system seemed an argument of some weight against the withholding of such agents. In retrospect one could consider this a case of severe pneumonia, beautifully described, during which acute glomerulonephritis developed with primitive chemical test suggesting elevated urea and anemia with partial remission. The affect of the therapy on the disease processes remain of questionable significance considering standards of therapy of today.

Such was the salutary experience of Robert Christison employing some of the therapeutic agents available to physicians in 1836 Bleeding, tartar emetic, calomel, opium, leeches, digitalis squill, bitartrate of potasah, and mercury.

Pierre Rayer—Traite des Maladies des Reins—The
French Take on Therapy

Gabriel Richet has written on the place of Pierre Rayer as the founder of French Nephrology. Rayer had previously published an atlas and a two volume book on skin diseases as well as making the discovery that glanders was contagious and could infect man. His masterpiece on renal disease was initiated with an atlas which appeared in 1839 giving a description of many kinds of kidney pathology as well as careful description with a microscope of the urinary sediment including casts and crystals of quinine. Volume One of his two volume edition *Traite des Malade des Reins* sets forth critical analysis of urinary density and methods to study urine correlating with clinical material. The concluding chapter of Volume Two gives the first detailed History of Nephrology from Hippocrates until his own time. Rayer gives full credit to Richard Bright in 1827 for originally establishing the kidneys as the responsible factor in the development of dropsy, coagulable urine with granular kidneys. On the initial page of his chapter Nephrite Albumineuse in Volume 2 is a long footnote he debates with himself what the disease should be called, "it has been suggested that the affliction be called *Bright's disease*, and I would have been very inclined to adopt that name, which dedicates the discovery of this famous doctor, would it not have seemed preferable to me to give it a significant scientific name." Rayer was intimately acquainted with the English literature on renal disease including Richard Bright, whom he always refers to with respect, only gently criticizing some of his interpretations, as compared with a more abrasive approach to the other "English pathologists", Robert Christison, James C. Gregory from Scottland, Jonathan Osborne from Ireland whom he alternately praises or chastises depending upon his own evaluation. Rayer was equally acquainted with the writings of the physicians who preceeded Bright, William Charles Wells and John Blackall, who had seen some correlation between coagualable urine, dropsy and kidney disease. He praised Robert Christison for his analysis of serum for identifying urea and Hematosin but equally criticizes him for " bragging about the effect of the combination of Cream of Tarter and Digitalis" as a diuretic when his own experience dictates otherwise.

The Paris hospitals of the first half of the nineteenth century, Hotel Dieu established in 829, the Pitie, and the Charite where Rayer was Professor, became the focus of an eclectic form of medicine.

Recognizing Edinburgh as the leading international medical center of the late eighteenth century, and to which many of the English physicians attended contributed to the relatively monolithic patter of English medicine. In contrast the medical climate in Paris after the Revolution became an eclectic force able to encompass on the one hand the likes of F. J.V. Broussais who used no medications but relied on excessive bleeding and popularized the epidemic use of leeches in France that spread world wide. This is to be contrasted with the critical empiricists like Pierre Louis, the developer of the *methode numerique,* a statistical method that questioned the use of blood letting in inflammatory diseases. (Louis was a favorite of William Osler who paid a visit to his grave in the early twentieth century and wrote a biographic chapter on him in *An Alabama Student).*

What will be the therapeutic spectrum of Pierre Rayer, the founder of French Nephrology, recognizing the contribution of Richard Bright just a little more than a decade after his establishing the clinical triad of coagulable urine, dropsy and diseased kidneys? Will he follow the English physicians in their use of bleeding, Dover powder (opium and Ipecac) and James powder (antimony trioxide and calcium dibasic phosphate), etc, (learned at Edinburgh) or take the critical empiricists' course of Louis, or relieve his patients of their blood to be caught up in the revolution of Broussais?

Let us start with a typical example of the management of one of Rayer's patients :

Obs. 2 (case summary) Exposure to cold and dampness.—Albuminous nephritis with dropsy. Cure by bleeding rest and light decoction of horseradish (used as a tea, often cultivated since antiquity and used by the Jews at Sedar service, having a biter pungent taste when scraped or bruised, having a diuretic effect, as well as being an expectorant, antiscorbutic (Boerhaave recommended it for scurvy). Reoccurence in 1839; pain in the renal region, cloudy sparse and strongly albuminous urine; complete cure after two months of treatment. (*Blood letting, gamboges, cream of tarter, colchicum wine*— Colchicum is a root from a plant grown in Asia Minor, (Colchus in Turkey) known since antiquity and known to be toxic with the well known effects of nausea, vomiting, diarrhea. Used for arthritis and effective even to day in gout. Also Couch-grass tea – *Ttiticum repens* is a pervasive perennial grass growing up to 1.5 m in many areas. Considered a soothing mild diuretic analgesic and antimicrobial used since the first century by Dioscorides, praised by Culpeper for use in kidney disease, even sick dogs eat it to relieve vomiting.

Rayer used a variety of teas, Mallow (gummy extract of roots of *Althaea officinalis*, marsh mallow. Used as a non-specific binding agent; as an emollient—a drug that reduces cohesion between particles of solid matter-+and demulcent—a lubricating agent—especially in cataplasms; and in drinks for patients with <u>renal colic,</u> and in enemas) Asparagus, (roots and shoots of *Asparagus officinalis*—a diuretic and aperient") of Senna (leaves of *Cassia acutifolia,* a diuretic and cathartic for which it is used today in view of its ability to irritate the colon); as well as Horseradish tea, Beargrape tea,

Juniper (Genievere) tea, Tea of Diuretic roots, Sparteine sulfate tea, etc

Triqueneaux, 33 years old, rather robust constitution, weaver, married, father of two children entered the Hospital of Charity on March 1, 1836. This man does not remember sickness other than small pox and that as a child. The dropsy from which he is suffering began three years ago; he had been working then for a year in Rheims in an extremely damp room, in which the earthen floor was below ground level; a room so cold that the heat of summer couldn't alleviate the humidity. He worked fourteen hours a day in this hole. He entered the hospital and stayed there for three weeks; he was cured by a Bitter—any bitter-tasting tonic drug that stimulates the appetite (ie an appetizer) by virtue of its local irritant action in the stomach – and diuretic wine: <u>then he went back to work in</u> <u>that same room for 11 months.</u>

On return the face is puffed, the thighs and especially the legs are swollen and retain the impression of a finger. His heart has its normal size; it makes no suspicious sound; the patient has no palpitations; he is not out of breath when he climbs stairs quickly, and he can run for a rather long time. Moreover, his pulse is rather strong (80 beats a minute) His skin is not feverish to the touch; his lungs sound perfect; the tongue normal, no excessive thirst, good appetite, good digestion, normal bowel movements, no abdominal pain, no fluctuation (succussion splash). His liver does not extend beyond the lower rib cage. The patient has never abused alcohol. He never had pain in the region of the kidneys.

His urine, pale and lemon color, treated alternatively with nitric acid and with heat result in a considerable precipitate of albumin.(Treatment: *12 ounces of blood removed, milk, couch-grass tea – Triticum repen.* Density of urine 1010, blood membranous, (having an buffy coat and other characteristics that signifies an inflammatory process) the patient confirms that he feels better, but there is no apparent change in his condition (Treatment: application of 20 leeches in the renal region), Manifests improvement.

Swelling in the legs has diminished, Triqueneaux assures us he has urinated more than in the preceding days and that is confirmed by the number of bottles he has filled up in 24 hours. On March 9 we prescribe a light horseradish tea (only the thick part of the root per pint). Urine much less dark containing mucus and albumin; swelling diminishes; by the 24th of March dropsy has completely disappeared. Continuance of the horseradish tea. He asks to leave and he is permitted to do so.

The dropsy has entirely disappeared; the face is in no way puffy;the legs show no signs of swelling, and the skin does not retain the indentation of a finger(doesn't pit); only the skin is plate and manifest this dull white tissue that has been bathed for a long time with serum or is saturated with it. The lungs, the heart, the digestive organs are functioning regularly; the patient feels strong and ready to go back to work.

I saw this man again on April 23, 1836; since leaving the hospital he had resumed his work as a weaver. It is several years later and Triqueneaux continues to be submitted to exposure to dampness, working in a very humid workshop, often tormented by thirst and drinking cold water; he has generalized edema, urine precipitates with very abundant flakes of albumin; (Treatment: 12 ounces of blood removed, 6 gr. of gamboges, whey with cream of tarter, food restricted to ¼ serving. Additional treatment: repeat blood removal, cream of tarter and restrict food, add colchicum wine— diarrhea produced. He develops pain in left kidney—

eight ounces of blood extracted by scarified cupping glasses applied at the point of pain. Complete disappearance of the pain. The patient leaves the hospital June 27, feeling better and cured of dropsy. The urine no longer contains even a trace of albumin. Ten days later, Triqueneaux came to see me to thank me for the care I had given him; his health had improved; the urine contained no more albumin."

Summary of therapy over a three year period: Bitters, Diuretic wine, Blood letting X 4, 20 leeches to renal area, Gambage, Cream of tarter, Restriction of diet, Colchicum wine, Couch tea and cupping. Except for the addition of the several teas, Colchicine and Horseradish treatment doesn't seem much different from that the English physicians (Bright didn't use leeches however). Etiology of the condition, exposure to cold and damp were similar. Alcohol was looked for carefully. Certainly Rayer was not over influenced by the *methode numerique* of Louis nor did he succumb to the excessive leech and blood letting of Broussais. Certainly Triqueneaux and his urine were carefully examined, the patient followed carefully and the results were favorable.

A less complex case follows which Rayer considered as an example of acute albuminous nephritis, with "a happy ending." Madam C...., Spanish, very strong constitution, abundant menstrual flow, after which having been exposed to cold and dampness, experienced, at the beginning of February 1833, a sluggishness, a kind of heaviness in the kidney region and legs which mad walking painful. At the same time her urine became reddish and formed abundant sediment; face was slightly puffy with edema of arms and legs and the urine contained a strong proportion of albumin. The patient took nitrated couch-grass tea (much like Triqueneau – Rayer was fond of teas in a variety or flavors and I have found over eleven different varieties previously noted. On the third day an impressive failure to eliminate the edema made bleeding necessary. Madame C… had some relief, but the edema remained stationary. With the use of horseradish begun in a dosage of a half ounce in a pint of water plus a bland diet the urine became much more abundant after a week, progressively less murky, less tinged with blood and finally less albuminous and the dropsy and concomitant conditions soon disappeared completely. Since that time Madame C… is enjoying a very good state of health an walks about without the least fatigue in the legs After the cure of the anasarca, Madame C… continued for a while with use of donkey milk without reoccurrence.

These two cases of acute Albuminous nephritis with recovery were in the minority of cases presented. In chronic Albuminous nephritis with complications Rayer "sadly reflected on the incurability of the illness" and recognized there often existed "no chance of for successful treatment" He concludes his summary of the therapeutic options available with a very conservative and reasoned approach that must have been the model for Sir William Osler's recommendation fifty two years later in treating renal disease in Osler's *Principles and Practice of Medicine* of 1892.

Rayer: "With the help of hygienic care of course, the physician will succeed, in some cases in removing secondary complications and in remediating, in part, the progressive deterioration of the constitution. To that end the doctor will recommend living in a dry and temperate in a dry and temperate environment, in a flat with southern exposure; proper alimentation appropriate to the digestive system, daily use of ferrouginous (iron) preparations, and a small quantity of good white wine. (Osler omits the wine) And in the case where, later the dropsy will disappear, where the disease is reduced to renal dysfunction or a disorder of urinary secretion, the patients could prolong their life by a continuation of the same regime, by habitual use of lukewarm aromatic baths, and by moderate exercise, if unfortunately the social class of most of them does not make it impossible to undergo costly and long term, continuous care."

However this approach doesn't limit Rayer in discussing later cases in a dizzying kaleidoscope array of therapeutic measures, many of which he condemns or finds of little use, but which depending upon the situation of the patient, he finds need to attempt to administer, not withstanding. In general the categories of available agents are similar to whose previously described by Bright, Christison and Osbourne.

"Among the successful remedies, (here Rayer is referring to established antiphlogistic measures in common use) one must put in first place, general blood letting and the application of cupping glasses in the lumbar region. In individuals of strong constitution, the amount of blood to be let should be in proportion to the rise in temperature and to the rapidity with which the dropsy has developed. And, according to whether or not the blood extracted from the vein appears more or less rich, if the clot is covered with a more or less abundant membrane, the blood letting should be repeated once or several times. In general, during that period of illness, by practicing blood letting, it is necessary to risk going beyond rather than remaining well within the limits that it seems necessary to attain" The vigorous use of blood letting was the norm on both sides of the English channel.

"When the spike in fever is less pronounced, the heat on the skin less intense, the constitution less strong, after an initial blood letting it is often preferable to have recourse to the application of cupping glasses on the lumber region. The application of leeches to the same region should be substituted for cupping glasses with pat6ients who are afraid of the use of the latter method, which, moreover, is much less painful than is generally thought in France."

Rayer recognized the complication of "phlegmonous erysipelas with the deep injection that is necessary to open a vein or application of cupping glasses or leeches and considered baths, emollients, (applying warmth and moisture) and of softening cataplasms (like a watery poultice, an external medicated application) often able to stop these inflammation at their outset."

Rayer recommends the patient stay in bed while fever persists, and encouraging perspiration by warm or steam baths, similar to Osbourne but without his enthusiastic reliance. Lukewarm drinks slightly nitrated with attention to keeping the body warm with suitable clothing such as flannel. Becoming more vigorous with treatment Rayer recommends "saline purgatives, especially if the patient is constipated ! Stronger purgative, such as Jalap root and Gamboge should be administered by preference in cases where the dropsy is considerable and when it has been little alleviated by blood letting." Then there is the remarkable statement, " The patients should drink as much as they want" The concept of the renal handling of water was not appreciated.

For gastrointestinal symptoms such as vomiting or diarrhea Rayer recommended warm baths, leeches on the anus, and small doses of opium. These three items are recommended together in one sentence, as if the middle item, leeches on the anus, were as benign and common as the two adjoining suggestions. Details on giving a bath include giving the bath near the bed, "so the he does not get cold in the trip from the bath to the bed. In cold weather especially patients should never be transported to the bathroom. When the baths are taken by convalescents it is preferable to gibe the baths in the evening shortly before sleep." These measures reflect the concern that a chill was a major factor as an etiological agent. Osbourne and others gave similar instructions.

Rayer considers next the treatment of chronic albuminous nephritis, suggesting that bleeding and scarified cupping (wet cupping to remove blood) be less vigorous, but the presence of fever or new onset edema or albuminuria warranted such treatment. Cauterization and setons (fistula tract often with a strip of sild or linen drawn through the sound to make an issue; ie, to keep it open.) to the renal area are described. Twelve drops of tincture of cantharis (or Cantharidis, beetle or Spanish fly usually applied as to the skin producing a blister. When used as a tincture for oral route it produced severe dysuria, abdominal pain, hematuria and even death. The mythology of its aphrodisicacal properties is related to its ability to irritate the lower urinary tract and produce a prolonged erection.) as well as balsamics and turpentine (both wood resin products, the popularity of balsamic as a dressing salad, originally promulgated from Moderna, Italy is a recent departure from its older therapeutic usages.) are suggested without firm recommendation. Mercury ointment applied to the skin is also given little recommendations. Sedlitz and Pullna water (both small towns in Bohemia with mineral springs), Cream of Tarter (potassium antimony tartrate) in Senna tea get higher marks as Rayer indicates, "one gets a noticeable reduction and sometimes a disappearance of the dropsy by purging the patient twice-a week with these agents."

Rayer continues to recommend the use of the GI tract to ameliorate fluid retention." The dropsy has sometimes diminished through the use of drastic purgatives, by administrating Elatruim (Bright's favorite purgative) Also recommended are Colocynth (a cathartic from the dried pulp of the unripe but full grown fruit of Citrellen colocynthus) mixed with extract of Henbane (hyoscyamus—an atropine like alkaloid) as well as Gambage (*gomme-gutte* a gum resin from an East India tree) or Scammonee (a plant native to eastern Mediterranean-a hydrogogue laxative.) Tincture of Colchicum is also mentioned for its effect in vomiting and purging. Ferruginous materials such as iron sulfate here added " when the patients are very weak." Rayer recognized and cautioned that" the resistance of the disease requiring a variation of trials, one can sometimes combine saline laxatives with drastic purgatives and bring about fatiguing disorder, followed by malaise and prostration."

Rayer continues in a conservative vein, The multiplicity of trials and variety of remedies (for dropsy) which have been successively recommended only indicate all to vividly the frequency of failure and difficulty of increasing in such cases, urinary secretion." Rayer agrees with Bright who "had little confidence in most diuretics" and then in a rebuke in a footnote, "Dr. Christison brags especially about the effects of the combined action of Cream of Tartar and digitalis." Rayer continues, stating that "Squill and digitalis rarely increase the urine in a measurably way and almost always result in upsetting the functions of the stomach. Tincture of squill and digitalis used as rubbing compounds on the body and limbs, have rarely appeared to me to have salubrious effects. These tinctures dirty the skin, the rubbing tires the patient, and is sometimes painful, when the skin is tightly stretched. Then again Rayer is more favorably impressed with wild horseradish tea indicating "that I have seen dropsy diminish and sometimes completely disappear through the use of wild horseradish tea."

There is an accompanying footnote to indicate that the dose needs to be increase and the root used which is less bitter and that caution needs to be taken that side effects of dyspepsia, nausea and desire to vomit are recognized, "as often happens rather frequently in chronic albuminous nephritis." Continuing in his appraisal of wild horseradish tea, Rayer indicates, "Several patients have refused to continue drinking that liquid because they find it disagreeable and it tires their stomach. I have seen others who, despite the perseverance with which they have used it have derived no relief from it. However, of all the diuretics, it is still the one which appears to me to have the greatest chance of success. (Previously discussed The Egyptians recognized horseradish as far back as 1500 B.C. While primarily used as a condiment today, it was recognized by the old herbalists as a diuretic among its other alleged uses, The prefix "horse" refers to its large size and coarseness – compare with horse chestnut – and "radish" from the Latin *radix* meaning root.)

Steam baths and diaphoretics are next considered by Rayer. In a footnote he gives recognition to Osborne (*On dropsies connected with suppressed perspiration and coagulable urine, 1835)* but is incredulous about Osborne's results of "curing 27 out of 36 with these methods. However he endorses water steam baths, which "have been used with success, not only for acute albuminous nephritis, but even for chronic albuminous nephritis." His staunchest criticism is leveled at the "English pathologist (who) generally recommend Dover powder (previously described on p.9)...as a powerful diaphoretic. James Powder passes also among them for a good diaphoretic; for my part, I feel myself obliged to declare that the trials I have made with these remedies in the treatment of dropsy stemming from chronic albuminous nephritis, have been almost completely unfruitful; rarely have these powders induced a salutary perspiration; and often the Dover's powder has been the occasion of malaise and desire to vomit (side effects of opium and ipecac if the doses is not adjusted). The diaphoresis that these remedies have produced in some cases, has had no or almost no advantageous influence on the progress of the dropsy" Is this judgment just the chauvinism of a proud Frenchman toward his "English pathologists" or astute clinical judgement from experience?

Chapter Six

Pulvis Ipecacunanhae et Opii—The Powder and the
Buccaneer Thomas Dover (1660 – 1742)

The most efficient diaphoretic is Dover's
Powder, 5-8 gr. 3 times a day with a warm bath.

Sir   Robert   Christison,   On   Granular
Degeneration of the Kidney, 1839, p. 65.

These are the several Symptoms of an
approaching Dropsy...The Thirst is more
intense, Urine less in Quantity, higher coloured,
coming near to the Water made in a Jaundice;
shortness of Breath to that Degree, that there is
no lying down in Bed; an Inability to all
Motions; a total loss of Appetite. The Legs,
thighs and all Parts of the Body, are full of
Water; which make up the frightful merciless
Retinue that attend this great Evil. Let me but
come to People as early in this Distemper, as
they generally apply for Relief from other
Physicians, and it shall be cured with as much

Certainty as any other Gentleman may cure a Distemper he thinks himself most Master of.

Thomas Dover, The Ancient Physician's Legacy to his Country, 6th Edition 1742, p.19-20, facsimile edition of Kenneth Dewhurst 1974.

Dover's powder, introduced in 1740, has been in the Pharmacopoeia for over 200 hundred years. It is usually considered a mixture of opium and ipecac and while originally prescribed as an antidote to the gout, has usually been considered as a sweating or diaphoretic agent. Sir William Osler, known as a therapeutic conservative, mentions the use of Dover's powder in his *Principles and Practice of Medicine*. In his chapter on typhoid fever, after initially promulgating his well known dictum, "The profession was long in learning that typhoid fever is not a disease to be treated mainly with drugs", Osler advocates Dover's powder, not as a diaphoretic agent but to counteract diarrhea. He also recommends its use for similar circumstances in tuberculosis, as well as in rheumatic fever to alleviate pain. Osler read a paper on Thomas Dover, *The Physician and Buccaneer* at the Johns Hopkins Historical Club in January 1895, which deals with Thomas Dover's career as a sea captain and buccaneer as well as his activities as a physician.

Dover was born in Barton-on-Heath, in the Cotswold, educated at both Oxford and Cambridge, took an apprenticeship with Thomas Sydenham. He was a fellow student with Hans Sloane, a less controversial figure and collector of art and other items that became the founding core of the British Museum, as well as becoming President of the Royal Society and the College of Physicians . Dover then settled in Bristol to begin his practice of medicine. At the age of forty-six he took to sea as a captain and doctor, in 1708 to raid Spanish settlements and capture Spanish ships. Bristol was the second largest seaport in England and famous for its expeditions to the New World. A group of merchants, including Dover who had a financial interest in the project, outfitted two ships, the *Duke* and the *Dutchess*. The project participated in many adventures, gathered considerable loot, as well as rescuing Alexander Selkerk, a Scotchman who had been stranded on a South Sea island for three and one half years and who became the model for Defoe's Robinson Crusoe. After three years at sea, having circumnavigated the globe Dover returned to England, much wealthier for his adventures and settled in London resuming his role as a physician.

In 1732 Dover wrote a popular book on medical treatment entitled *The Ancient Physician's Legacy to his Country*, having eight subsequent printings through 1771. On the title page is stated, an *Account of the several Diseases incident to Mankind; described in so plain a Manner, That any person may know the Nature of his own Disease together with the several Remedies for each distemper, faithfully set down. Designed for the use of all Private Families.* The book made a great commotion among the coffee houses of London, because it was primarily a manual for patient's use to treat their own diseases or *distempers*, as Dover calls them. The braggadocio of the old Buccaneer's style and his truculent manner of dealing with colleagues who disagreed with his methods contributed to the controversy. Perhaps the most over-the-top tale is his description of an epidemic of plague on board ship off the coast of South America.

> When I took by Storm the two Cities of Guaiaquil (Guayaquil- a city and port of Ecuador, currently the gateway to the Galapagos Island), under the Line, in the South Seas, it happen'd that not long before, the Plague had raged amongst them. For our better Security,

therefore, and keeping our People together, we
lay in their Churches, and likewise brought
thither the Plunder of the Cities: We were very
much annoy'd with the Smell of the dead
Bodies....In less than Forty-eight Hours we had
in our several Ships, one hundred and eighty
men in this miserable Condition. I order'd the
Surgeons to bleed them in both Arms, and to go
round to them all with Command to leave them
bleeding till all were blooded.... We had on
board Oil and Spirit of Vitriol (sulfuric acid)
sufficient, which I caused to be mixed with
Water to the Acidity of a lemon, and make them
drink very freely of it; so that notwithstanding
we had one hundred and eighty odd down in
this most fatal Distemper, yet we lost on more
than seven or eight; and even these owed their
Deaths to the strong Liquors which their Mess-
Mates procured for them.

While as we see Thomas Dover was a believer in
bleeding for anything that could be classified as
inflammation, as were all the doctors in his day, he also
employed quicksilver or metallic mercury with abandon.
He was often called the Quicksilver doctor. He scolded
his colleagues who employed blisters (application of
Cantharides, Spanish flies, or other agent that would
produce a blister as a counter irritant). Dover favored
the introduction of inoculation against smallpox and
opposed older treatments recommended by Paracelsus
such as bezoar stones and other outdated nostrums. He
was always respectful to his teacher, Sydenham
advocating relief of pain and cold baths for fever, but not
mentioning horseback riding which was one of
Sydenham's favorite remedies. Because Dover's doses of
narcotics were considered excessive his opponents
advised his patients to prepare their wills before
consulting him. However Dover countered with tales of

wondrous lightening-like cures, with letters from gratified patients to back up his claims for cures for everything from the gout to the dropsy. It is in this book, *The Ancient Physicians Legacy* on page 14 as the third remedy for gout, not the first, that the famous prescription for the preparation of his powder is set forth.

Take Opium one Ounce, Salt-Petre and Tartar vitriolated, each four Ounces Ipocacuana one Ounce, Liquorish one Ounce. Put the Salt-Petre and Tartar into a red hot Mortar, stirring when with a Spoon till they have done flaming,- Then powder them very fine; after that slice in your Opium; grind these to a Powder, and then mix the other Powders with these. Dose from forty to sixty or seventy Grains in a Glass of White-Wine Posset, going to bed.- Covering up warm, and drinking a Quart or three pints of the Posset-Drink while sweating."

Dover continues describing the expected effects of his Powder on the gout. "In two or three Hours, at farthest, the Patient will be perfectly free from Pain: and though before not able to put one Foot to the Ground, 'tis very much if he cannot walk the next Day." Thomas Dover continues commenting on criticism of others concerning the dose of Opiates," Some Apothecaries have desired their Patients to make their Wills, and settle their Affairs, before they venture upon so large a Dose as I have recommended, which is from Forty to Seventy Grains. As monstrous as they may represent this, I can produce undeniable Proofs, where a Patient of mine has taken to no less a Quantity than an Hundred Grains, and yet has appear'd abroad the next Day." As to why this high dose is well tolerated, Dover had a suggestion, " This Notion of theirs (that a high dose is detrimental) proceeds entirely from their Ignorance, and from the Want of knowing the Nature of those Ingredients that are mix'd up with it, for they naturally weaken the Power of the Opium."

Let us examine the composition of Dover's powder more carefully. The first ingredient Opium, one Ounce was as well known and appreciated then as today. Poppy, Papaver sominiferum grown extensively in many countries of Europe and Asia as well as America, reaches a height of 2-3 feet with seeds and flowers of various colors. It is the dried seeds producing a milky extract of various alkaloids, morphine, codeine, papaverine, etc. that is obtained from the dried material. Opium has a long and well known history from Assyrian times to the Opium Wars of the 19th century, and in works of literature as well. Opium is primarily a pain reliever, blocking the opium receptors of the brain but useful in diarrhea. It was probably the major factor in the relief of Dover's patient with gout, relieving his pain "in two to three hours, at the farthest (to) be perfectly free from pain; and though before not able to put one foot to the ground, 'tis very much if he cannot walk the next day." It is doubtful if it had any direct or long lasting effect on the gout itself. In fact Dover goes on to plug "Mynsycht's Elixir of Vitriol taken in large quantities most certainly destroys gouty matter; yet for some time it may cause pain; but taken in its due latitude, if water will quench fire it must in the end have its desired effects." Mynsycht's Elixir of Vitriol, Acid vitrioli aromaticaticum, is sulfuric acid in wine, introduced by Adrian Mynsycht in 1631, the formula including many other aromatics as well. Opium can produce sweating or diaphoresis by increasing peripheral blood flow. Such effects were to become the powder's chief usage. These properties were attributed to Dover's powder by later observers as well as by Dover himself. The "covering up warm, and drinking a quart or three pints of the Posset-Drink while sweating" may have been an added significant effect, as well.

Next let us consider the Salt-Petre and Tartar vitriolated, each four Ounces which I will consider as filler agents. Salt-Petre or Sal Nitre is potassium nitrate and Tartar vitriolated is Kali sulphuratum or potassium sulfate, adding some grittiness to the overall mechanical effect of the powder.

Next comes Ipocacuana, one Ounce. Ipecacuanha comes from the root of a small shrub like plant grown in Brazil. The name of the plant reflects the Portuguese native word, i-pe-kaa-guene which means "road-side sick-making plant" reflecting the ability to induce vomiting by its primary ingredient, Emetine. The chief ingredients of ipecac are the alkaloids Emetine, cephaelin and Psychotrine. 1.5 to 2% of the bark contains these alkaloids of which Emetine is the major component. At low doses ¼ to 2 grains Ipecac is an expectorant and diaphoretic but at larger doses, 15 to 20 grains, the more familiar effect of vomiting is predominant.

The next element in Dover's powder is Liquorish, one ounce. Licorice is also a root of the plant, Glycerrihiza glaba. It has a sweat taste and mildly cathartic. It is often included in Chinese herb mixtures and was known in the ancient world and grows widely. King Tutankhamen was even buried with a supply. The sweetness of the material is related to glycyrrhizic acid, a compound with two sugars attached to a steroid-like molecule. It has been known that glycyrrhizic can support patients with adrenal insufficiency, but it wasn't recognized until relatively recently that it modulates the 11 beta hydroxy-dehydrogenase, decreasing the degradation of cortisol. The similarity of the structure of glycyrrhetic acid to that of steroids may also contribute to its cortisol effect. Licorice finds its usage not only as a sweet agent in candy but as flavoring agents in tobacco, soft drinks, in cough syrup and in medicines to mask their bitter taste.

The latter effect is the one Thomas Dover employed in his famous powder to mask the otherwise bitter mixture.

And what about the White wine Posset? A Posset is milk curdled with beer, wine or other liquor. A typical Posset is a mixture of 2 parts small beer and one part milk. Undoubtedly the alcohol was a contributing factor to the salutary effect experienced with Dover's patient in gout.

The major ingredients in Dover's powder are opium and ipecac. One ounce of each or 30 grams in a total of 11 ounces or 330 grams of the entire mixture. Let us consider the opium first and making some assumptions such as the amount of the active ingredient morphine being about 10 % of the total opium. Now noting Dover's prescription of a "dose from forty to sixty to seventy grains in a glass of white-wine posset, going to bed" it is calculated that about 0.36 grains (5.40 mg) of morphine to be present in the forty grain dosage and that in the seventy grain dose would contain 0.63 grains (9.5 mg) morphine. Opium contains additional alkaloids other than morphine that might increase its potency, but taking the mixture orally would reduce its immediate effectiveness. Certainly a potent dose of a narcotic, but not an excessive dose of opium that would hardly warrant his opponents recommending that the recipients write out their wills before taking Dover's powder. The same sort of assumptions can apply to the ipecacuanha root. The 40 grain dose would contain about 3.6 grains of ipecac and the 70 grain dose about 6.3 grains of ipecac. Both of these dosages would contain what is considered a low dose, 0.25 to 2.0 grains enough to result in sweating or expectoration. Larger doses of 15 to 30 grains have the more familiar emetic function.

One of the striking features of this Dover's Powder is the absence of a single potent cathartic in the mixture, which was usually present in the nostrums of the day. I considered that double dose of potassium containing drugs, Salt Petre (potassium nitrate) and Tartar Vitrioated (potassium sulfate) might lead to potassium intoxication, but calculation suggests that it was not an excessive amount. The avoidance of a high dose of ipecac, minimizing vomiting but promoting the sudorific aspects of the mixture, was either a point of pharmacological insight or a piece of good luck. The opium and the ipecac acted in concert to produce this effect as a sweating agent, so important in the later use of the powder. It was probably serendipidity that combined a low dose of ipecac and a hefty dose of opium, at least enough to cure the patient's acute gouty distemper, rather than have to experiment with a controlled drug trial. And how about that parting touch with the use of that sweet Liqouirsh to make the powder palatable? Its bitterness without the Liquorish might not have sold so well. It adds up to a masterful stroke for patients and the medical profession.

The preparation of   Dover's powder is rather challenging for anyone, including an apothecary. The salt-petre and tartar vitriolated are "put into a red-hot mortar, stirring them with a spoon till they have done flaming, then powdered fine." How many homes then or today have that "red hot mortar" available? Then the opium is sliced in, ground to a powder and then mixed with the other powder. Even our contemporary pharmacist might struggle with its preparation, especially arranging for that "red hot mortar" and all that "stirring with a spoon till they have done flaming" and grinding to a powder, shaving and mixing. Certainly this is not the usual off the shelf prescription we are accustomed to see our pharmacists prepare.

Dower was certainly very familiar with the clinical presentation of gout for which his powder was to alleviate. The following extended description may serve to remind contemporary physicians what gout was like in the early eighteenth century.

A regular gout may most properly be term'd Podagra, because it begins in the first joint of the great toe, and usually about midnight; where, after it has rack'd the patient forty-eight hours with a violent fixed pain, a small tumour begins to appear, increasing gradually; after that, an inflammation, and then the violence of the pain abates.

The first fit may last a fortnight, or three weeks; but a great weakness and tenderness in the part afflicted, remains much longer.

The patient may feel no more of this disease for two or three years, or at soonest a twelvemonth: but what adds much to the misfortune of this distemper, is, that every fit becomes more painful, and the paroxysms more frequent and lasting.

The gouty matter increasing, rises to the ankles and knees, which, as was said before, swell with inflammation: This degree of the distemper, by some authors is called Morbus Articularis, and is always attended with asymptomatical fever; for as the pain wears off, the fever abates.

Thus it takes its progress, increasing by degrees, till the poor patient is lacerated, and torn to pieces; chalk-stones working out of the joints, attended with other melancholy circumstances.

It must be observed, towards the latter end of this disease, when the fluids are almost wholly changed into gouty matter, the fits are not so regular, nor the pains so violent; but then the patient is seldom free from them.

Thomas Dower's description of diseases in his Physician's Legacy to his Country is usually not as vividly drawn, but his familiarity with gout, as well as compassion toward the patient is apparent in this description. He goes on to consider therapy. "There have been so many unsuccessful attempt made to alter this disease, that patients have very little faith left, and (as they commonly say) have no hopes from any thing but patience and warm flannel....Notwithstanding the many fruitless attempts that have been made to cure this miserable distemper, providence has in this, as well as in all other diseases, left means for recovery, which in many instances I am able to make appear." His confidence and braggadocio make their appearance here. "I shall refer to one (cure), where the curious may be satisfied: The coachman of the right honourable the Lord Viscount St. John had a long and tedious fit of the gout, and was hardly able to stir without crutches; I gave him a very pleasant easy Sudorific (not further characterized); which had its desired effect: - Insomuch that the day following, he walked from Albemarle-street to Cecil-street, to give me thanks. He came to me without the help of a stick and with strait shoes on: the swelling was entirely gone: he affirmed that he was never better in his life; and that he as able to walk from one end of the town to the other. This is about twenty–five Years ago." Now this was an appreciative patient!

That "pleasant easy Sudorific" not further characterized was the first prescription recommended for the gout by Dover. The second prescription "without Opiates, or painful remedies which I am a stranger to and very much dislike" follows:

Take Tamarinds half an ounce, leaves of Senna two drams, Rheuberb one dram, boil them in water to three ounces; strain them off, and dissove in them of manna and the purging syrup of roses, each one ounce syrup of

buck-thorn and Elixer Proprietatis, each two drams.—
Drinking Posset-Drink, or thin gruel between motion,—
taking this once or twice a week will lessen the gouty
matter, and break the force of the fit.

Tamarinds is a large tree from India with multiple
alleged pharmacological usages including as a cathartic.
Senna is a small shrub. The name is Arabian and its
leaves are known for purgative action. The tea is popular
today. Rheuberb also a mild cathartic from the root of a
common garden plant. Manna, probably not the manna
or bread from the bible but the resin from *Fraxinus ornus*,
is again a weak cathartic from which mannose and
mannital were first isolated. Buckthorn, has berries that
are a strong cathartic. Elixer Proprietatis (Paracelsi)
referring to Paracelsus's own elixir, from the inspissated
juice of aloe, from Arabian sea, used as a cathartic today.

While Dover recommends that "taking this once or twice
a week, will lessen the gouty matter and break the force
of the fits", it is certainly plainly evident that this fourth
prescription for gout is nothing but a mixture of
laxatives having this as its primary purpose.

It was the third prescription of Thomas Dover to
improve gout, Pulvis Ipecacunanhae et Opii that
remained in the Pharmacopoeia for over 200 years. Its
unique combination of opium and ipecac became
popular as a diaphoretic agent and later, as with William
Osler, as an agent for relief of diarrhea along with a host
of other presumed usages. Kenneth Dewhurst in his
Thomas Dover's Life and Legacy, indicates that "After
Dover's death it (the powder) was appropriated by the
quack Joshua Ward who popularized it as a sweating
powder. After Wards death his recipe book was found
to contain details of two powders, one identical with
Dover's recipe, and the other with the addition of white
hellebore (root of the white hellebore, *Veratrum viride*, an

emetic containing several alkaloids). This plagiarism probably saved Dover's powder from passing into obscurity, and certainly led to its inclusion in the London Pharmacopoeia of 1788." This was forty six years after his heath in 1735 and fifty six years after the publication of the first edition of the *Ancient Physician's legacy to his Country* in 1732. Dover probably would have been surprised by the acclaim later generation would apply to his powder, since during his life time his use of mercury was his defining attribute, since he was known as the "quicksilver doctor."

Roy Porter in his *The Greatest Benefits to Mankind* in his chapter on the Enlightenment indicates that " The eighteenth century has been dubbed the golden age of quackery (an obscure term that may have come from the Dutch 'quacksalver' or quicksilver doctor)." Quacks included such people as Mesmer, with his magnets, James Grahman a Scot who advocated mud bathing and the electrified Celestial Bed, as well as Joshua Ward (1685-1761). He made a fortune out of his "pill and drop", antimony, an antipyretic and an emetic and the "drop" being a vigorous purgative having multiple effects, as well as his recipe book perpetuating Dover's powder as a sweating agent.

Dover's Powder was well received by the community of physicians. While its use as an agent in gout was disappointing, its use as a depletion therapy, especially to encourage sweating, took hold. "The age-old medical regimes: blood-letting, sweating, purging, vomiting and other ways of expelling bad humours had a hold upon the popular imagination and reflected medical confidence in such matters." J. Worth Estes in *Hospital Life in Enlightenment Scotland* traces Dr. Andrew Duncan's, Sr. attendance and use of medication on the teaching ward of the Royal Infirmary of Edinburgh in 1795.

Phyllis V. age 42 was admitted to the infirmary with a diagnosis of diabetes mellitus with polydipsia, polyphagia, and massive polyuria. Initally the patient was treated with alum to decrease excessive urine output, then Cinchona, presumably for the same reason, blistering, on day 15. An emetic and a cathartic to strengthen the patient's stomach and relax her bowels. Since the urine output remained high, cold water compresses were applied over the kidneys followed by electricity over the kidneys. "She was still spilling excess sugar into her urine, as determined by tasting it!" She then developed signs of a respiratory infection and was treated with similar agents. " He also prescribed Dover's powder as a diaphoretic to help remove the fever." After additional treatments including dilute solution of cantharides orally, lime water, urine out put stabilized at less that five pounds per day (2400 ml) and after six months in the hospital she was discharged.

The difficulties of treating diabetes before insulin are apparent and Dover's powder became one of the mélange of medications commonly used at that period.

Richard Bright at Guy's Hospital in London, reported in 1827 on the triad of dropsy, coagulable urine and abnormal granular kidneys. While his list of medications include many of the agents popular in the day, similar to those at the Royal Infirmary of Edinburgh, from where he received his medical degree, Dower's powder was not one of his favorite choices. However Case 1, John King did received some of the components: Sumat Mist. effervese. cum Vini Ipecacuanhae, Olei Ricini cum Tinct. Opii. The ipecac, and opium are there as well as caster oil, but not according to the specifications of Dover.

A more enthusiastic proponent would be Johnathan Osborne of Dublin who following the lead of Bright confirmed much of his findings in a slim volume entitled *On the Nature and Treatment of Dropsical Diseases,* 1833. He was much impressed by the finding of "suppressed perspiration" as a major cause of this form of renal disease. He vigorously employed warm baths of every source, along with Dover's powder, reporting remarkable improvement in patient's general condition. "When a patient was placed under my care with general edema coagulable urine and dry skin, I direct him to be kept in bed, in order to maintain warmth of the surface…The first medication is a purgative followed by a foot bath, hip bath, or general bath, water or vapor at night with *Pulvi Ipeac with Opio.*" Four of his six reported cases received warm baths and *Pulvi. Doveri.*

Another follower of Richard Bright was Robert Christian of Edinburgh who likewise confirmed Bright's observation and in 1829 and 1839 and declared, " the most efficient diaphoretic is Dover's powder with a warm bath." He employed the powder in the management of many of his cases.

No one can question the propriety of the diaphoretic method of cure of the primary disease.The most efficient diaphoretic is Dover's powder which should always be conjoined with the warm bath. No other remedy gives more relief…so that its ultimate good effects can be scarcely be doubted. It commonly occasions sweating for some time afterwards and is followed by quiet sleep. Dover's powder is preferable to (Acetate of ammonium) being scarcely less useful as an anodyne and calmitive for removing pain and allaying irritability and restlessness.

Such were the accolades provided by Robert Christian for the treatment of granular degeneration, his name for the condition described by Bright several years earlier. Note how Dover's Powder is praised as an complement to warm baths as a diaphoretic agent, but also by virtue of it containing opium, as calming and analgesic agent, reinforcing the original use of the powder as a treatment for gout. And yet of the thirty one cases presented by Christian only five received the powder. This may be explained by Christian's later reservation about the enthusiastic results of Osborne." I sincerely wish that my experience of the effects of the diaphoretic plan could bear out the very sanguine encomiums bestowed upon it by Dr. Osborne.... I have several time seen general perspiration both spontaneous and from the use of diaphoretics fail to produce any material relief. Still no one can question the general propriety of the diphoretic method of cure. "

On the other hand, Pierre Rayer considered the founder of French Nephrology, while recommending warm baths and perspiration, eschewed the use of Dover's powder. In his *Traite des Maladies des Reins et des Alterations de la Secretion Urinaire* while favoring wild horseradish tea as a diuretic, and recommending warm baths, the "English Pathologists" recommendation for Dover's powder comes in for some rebuke.

"A few successes resulting from steam baths in the treatment of this dropsy have naturally led to trying diaphoretics and several agents which have a remarkable influence on the functioning of the skin. The well-known relationship between the functions of the skin and the urinary functions seem to fortify the hopes that are most rarely realized.

English pathologists generally recommend Dover's powder, repeated three times a day as a powerful diaphoretic. James Powder (Antimony calcium phosphate) passes among them for a good diaphoretic; for my part, I feel myself obliged to declare that the trials I have made with these remedies in the treatment of dropsy stemming from chronic albuminous nephritis, have been almost completely unfruitful; rarely have these powders induced a salutary perspiration and often the Dower's powder has been the occasion of malaise and the desire to vomit. The diaphoresis, that these remedies have produced in some cases, has had no or almost no advantageous influence on the progress of the dropsy.

Rayer may not have incorporated Dover's balanced mixture of opium and ipecac, as originally recommended, avoiding the emetic effect of the later and the "malaise" of the former. He was very familiar with the reports of Bright, as well with the studies of Jonathan Osborne in Ireland on the effect of perspiration induced with baths and Dover's powder   At this point Rayer commenting on Jonathan Osborne in *On dropsies connected with suppressed perspiration and coagulable urine, London, 18 35,* "Doctor Osborne is said to have cured 27 patients out of 36 (remarkable result if, among these cases, there were not a lot of acute cases), following a method which is in reality only the joining of the most recommended of means (blood letting, cupping glasses, purgatives, simple baths, steam baths, sudorifics, vesicatories, etc.) but what he uses with a particular view in mind, that of reestablishing cutaneous perspiration which (he believes) is almost always suppressed in this disease. Dr. Osborne explains the salutary effects of these remedies, of bleeding, even of vesicatories, by diaphoresis."   Here Rayer seems to cast doubt on the results of Osborne as well as on the effectiveness of sweating, as applied to Dover's powder in the ability to modify the underlying disease process.

SUMMARY

Thomas Dover followed his apprenticeship with Sydenham with a tour of duty as a sea captain before settling down to the practice of medicine. His swashbuckling style flavored his medical writing in his *The Ancient Physician's Legacy to his Country,* with tales of adventure as "when (he) took by storm the two Cities of Guaiaquil" during the plague epidemic. While respectful of the teachings of his mentor, Sydenham, favoring cold baths and comforting the patient, he was equally vehement in deprecating those who followed the older methods of Paracelsus or advocated blistering. "An eminent Physician was ask'd, How Blistering came so much in Fashion? He answer'd they had it from the Indians. <u>But I, that have seen more Indians than all the Physicians in England deny that the Indians ever make use of Blisters.</u> They do often cauterize; and in all Fevers amongst them, they cover the Patients over in the Sand till they are in profuse Sweat, and then throw them into cold Water; by which Means they become well." The use of cold water may be a tribute to his mentor, Sydenham.

Dover's powder, his third attempt to cure gout, became his one claim to immortality with his buccaneering exploits in the background. Wonderfully designed to contain just the right dose of opium to give relief from pain and providing some diaphoretic effect, it avoided a high dose of ipecac that would have produced vomiting yet preserving its alleged diaphoretic action (Rayer's experience with the Powder causing vomiting and malaise to the contrary). The Powder was tastefully seasoned with a dash of Liquorish to mask the bitter taste, combined with fillers to improve the mechanical feel of the powder. The preparation went on to be serviceable as a diaphoretic and as with many other medication, to have alternative or off-label uses as well. The dose of Opium was always welcome as an analgesic or to counter diarrhea as with William Osler almost two hundred years later. Of course the white Poset wine used as a chaser in the original prescription for gout was a nice touch. But was Dover's powder alone really that effective as a diaphoretic or was it all those warm baths and heavy blankets and white wine Posset that did the trick? Was Pierre Rayer's condemnation of Dover's powder just a proud Frenchman's rebuttal to the "English pathologist" or were his observations cogent?

Chapter Seven

A Conversation Between Two Leeches Concerning
Round Worms: Their History, Function, and
Contribution to Medical Therapy—Past and Present

"In the 18th century, punctuation marks were as common
as medicinal leeches
and just about as scientific."

Participants:

Leech #1   older scholarly type
Leech #2   enthusiastic neophyte

Leech #2   We are back, did you hear?

Leech #1   What do you mean back? We have always been a glorious partner in medical therapy. Even in ancient Egypt our blood sucking ancestors were a favorite to cure everything from A to Z. Our portraits are on the tombs of the pharaohs. We are even mentioned in Proverbs, 30, 15: "The leech (alukah) has two daughters..."

Leech #2   Yes, and my Professor tells me that we appear in literature as well.

Leech #1   Right. Even the Bard has recognized us.

Leech #2   Shakespeare ends his *Timon of Athens*, "Bring me into your city, And I will use the olive with my sword, Make war breed peace, and make peace stint war, make each Prescribe to other, as each other's leech. Let our drums strike."

Leech #1   For a young leech you are really into old literature. But that us of "leech" is from the Middle English meaning a doctor or physician. The word leech is from Anglo-Saxon, loece, meaning to heal which is in reference to a Doctor, as used by Shakespeare at the end of Timon of Athens. That's because i9n those days the docs and our ancestors were thought of in the same breath whenever bloodletting was needed. The French have a less harsh sounding word, Sangsue, meaning bloodsucker (sang-sucer). Isn't that a more mellifluous and appropriate? But the British have a better example from their literature in William Wordsworth 's poem. *"Resolution and Independence"*, about the lonely Leech-gather on the Moor: "He told, that to these waters he had come to gather leeches, being old and poor: Employment hazardous and wearisome! And in this way he gained an honest maintenance"...(stanza X V)

Leech #2   I don't care about that poor leech gather. What about us?

Leech #1   May I continue with Wordsworth? "From pound to pond he roamed, from moor to moor;

Housing, with God's good help, by choice or chance And in this way he gained an honest maintenance... Gathering leeches, far and wide, He traveled; stirring thus about his feet The waters of the pools where they abide."

Leech #2   "They abide." He is talking about where we live now.

Leech # 1   Will you let me finish? (Leech # 2 shakes his head OK) Well then: "Once I could meet with them on every side; But they have dwindled along by slow decay; Yet still I preserve, and find them where I may" (Stanza XVll)

Leech #2   Wordsworth is partial to that leech gatherer. But think of us poor leeches, "dwindled long by poor decay" . We need some other poet to tell our side of the story.

Leech #1   Literary references may satisfy some but we are God's gift to the doctor. We are always here when his pills, tincture and advice fail.

Leach #2   But look here (showing the Wall street Journal and Baltimore Sun articles) You are behind the times. We made an appearance on the very first page of the Wall Street Journal   December 27, 2004 in their expose on the ridiculously high cost of medical care. There we are in bold letters right under the headline, Leeches $ 81 each. We do are work much cheaper than all those trumped up hospital charges. And a more recent article in the prestigious Baltimore Sun of 1/23/11 is entitled *Leeches Making a Come Back* with pictures of us art work. You know sucking out a big hematoma the Plastic Surgeons had made.

Leech #1   You know we don't have to be picked up in some back yard pond anymore. The ponds in France and England, like that one described by Wordsworth were just about fished out. But Biopharm in Hendy, South Wales has created a leech farm supplying *hirudo medicinalis*, that is us, bred in a sterile, pure environment, with ultraviolet light sterilization and reverse osmosis insuring the hightest clinical standards, We can be delivered anywhere around the World with an E-mail.

Leech #2   And I have heard of an even closer modern leech farm, Leeches USA, LTD, in Westbury, N.Y. for the local crowd. They advertise on the internet. They give careful instructions on our care and use. And the price is right. Not that over inflated $81 dollars, only $7.50 each, with slight charge for shipping.

Leech #1   We are worth every penny of it. Consider the high cost of breeding us in fresh water pools, transporting us and keeping us in the pharmacy awaiting a call to action.

Leech #2   But your are not listening to me. The reason we made the Wall Street Journal and the Baltimore Sun is that the docs are beginning to employ our services again. Imagine it. We were just about put out of business in the middle of the nineteenth century. We are back in action taking care of the nasty hematomas that are beyond the shill of the plastic surgeons. We are now doing a "leech debridement", just as in the glory days of the early nineteenth century when any doctor that was worth his salt, worldwide, relied on our *"slow by sure"* method of bold letting to cure the patient.

Leech #1   Don't you know the story of your come back to grace. We had an image problem. But now we are mother's little helper. It was back about fifteen years ago when a surgeon, Joseph Upton, having taken many hours to sew a 5 year old ear back on, after a dog had bitten it off, it was noted that the newly attached area was beginning to swell and become congested with dark venous blood.

Leech # 2   That is when he thought of us. Leeches to the rescue! A dozen of us placed on the area in no time had the dark stagnant hematoma sucked up and the area looking hunky dory again.

Leech #1   Didn't your History Professor tell you about that famous French doctor, Pierre Rayer, the one who wrote *Traite des Reins* ("Treatise on the Kidneys" - but that is way back in 1839) in our glory days in the early nineteenth century when we were an important part of the doctor's therapeutic basket of tricks for almost every difficult chore. Remember they didn't have Penicillin, laser therapy or any of that junk at that time. Well this Rayer in his book describes how his patient Marie Roux, 26 years old of strong constitution who had edema of the legs, shortness of breath and pain in the lumbar area was cured by the application of several of our ancestors, doing what comes naturally to them, doing a leech phlebotomy, which fixed her up.

Leech #2   Your are right, my History Professor told us about those glory days. But now we ar back in operation today helping out the plastic surgeons, evacuating nasty hematomas developing after any procedures. He also told us that modern day doctors have in addition figured out how to chemically synthesize our unique and superior Heparin for those allergic to it. We use it of course to make the blood we suck up more liquid and easier to get at. Only imagine they have the nerve to call our produce Hirudin and even bottle it as a substitute for those allergic to Heparin, not even giving us credit for its first time use. They manufacture it as an anticoagulant and deprived us of the royalties.

Leech #1   But of course we have no need for money. We have no expenses   nor pockets to put the money in.

Leech #2   Modern biochemists have not only isolated Hirudin   from our salivary glands but a hyaluronidase. (aside) That is an enzyme that breads down tissue like our substance that increases the permeability at the site of our attack. Also they have isolated a histamine –like vasodilator and a thing they cal Calgin that prevents the bite from clotting off and interruption our work.   It also makes the bite less painful. Not only that but sometimes bite may cause an infection and we carry with us a bug for this purpose, Aeromonas hydrophial which lives in out gut and allows to give the recipient a parting shot. That same bug helps us digest the blood we suck up . It sort of does double duty for us.

Leech #1   My, your Professor has taught you so much! Well all that is interesting and I knew we would be back on the medical stage soon again especially after the great days we had in the past. Did you know that the word *leech* is from the Anglo Saxon word *Loece*-meaning to heal and that it is synonymous with Doctor, as used when I quoted earlier   Shakespeare use of leech at the end of Timon of Athens. That's because in those days the docs and our ancestors were thought of in the same breath, when ever blood letting was needed, and blood letting was their Magic bullet or so they thought. The French have a more appropriate and less harsh sounding monosyllabic utterance for us, ie: *Sangsue,* meaning blood (sang). Isn't that s more mellifluous and appropriate?

Leech #2   I guess your are going to tell me about that French doctor with the tree first names, Francois-Joseph-Victor   Broussais, the doctor in Napolean's Grande Armee who was our most illustrious and greatest advocate?

Leech #1   That is right. He was born on December 17, 1772 in Saint-Malo. As you mentioned he was a military surgeon with Napolean.   He was among many physicians of that time who jumped on the inflammation (aside- from *inflammo* to inflame or burn) band wagon, an old concept of the ancients where heat, redness and swelling suggested the accumulation of blood in one or another part of the body.   To counteract this inflammation the ancients had used blood letting. That is where we come in.

Leech #2   Is that the same thing as the inflammation we have today?

Leech #1   More or less but today the doc's definition of inflammation is more scientific and not as gross. But let me continue. As with everything concerning   the   Ancients,   especially   the   Greeks, moderation was the motto and blood letting was employed on a limited basis. However it was getting out of hand by the early nineteenth century, considered as a physician's cure-all. Supplementing these measures laxatives, diuretics, cupping and sweating agents were in addition employed in generous quantity. Broussais revived the old idea that using our help would simplify the blood letting procedure, avoiding the need for opening a vein that might get infected and suppurate.

Leech #2   Broussais had the right idea of using our help in the thing we do best.

Leech #1   That is right and it would represent a painless blood-letting that would do the trick just as well as phlebotomy or in conjunction with it as a sort of double whammy.

Leech #2   Sounds like that man Broussais sized us up just right for the job.

Leech #1   And Broussais had the screwy notion, obtained from his autopsy experience that blood was often found in the mucus membranes of the gastrointestinal tract. This excessive blood in the GI tract he figured was the culprit for this and a bunch of other ailements. It was a kind of a gastroenteritis that could be cured by the removal of blood by the efforts of our ancestors.

Leech #2   And that is where we come in. Leeches were applied to the, imagine it, to the rectum and anywhere else as well, so that we could unload the blood, reduce the inflammation. That idea of our sucking away at some poor fellow's rectum sounds gross with regard to the victim, excuse me, I mean patient, but I understand it was the thing to do. One of my old Professors had us look up a Jonathan Osborne (aside— an Irish physician and follower of Richard Bright, the one who gave his name to kidney disease)

Leech #1   There you go quoting your old Professor again. This time I am up with you. I know that article *On the Nature and Treatment of Dropsical Diseases,* 1834 and on page 57 where there is recorded in a footnote, "In the Dublin Medical Journal I have described a convenient mode of introducing leeches into the rectum by securing them with silk threads attached to the groves of an instrument prepared for the purpose."

Leech #2   Yea, that must have been hard on us being tied by a tread in that strange environment and think of the patient having to suffer us in this location. And think about our being in so an unnatural dark place. But now we have had a revival of interest in our buddies performing limited duty in plastic surgical procedures, rather than fighting inflammation with that outworn idea of bleeding.

Leech #1   Has your Professor told you about the more recent   article by Dr. Granzow entitled *Simple method for control of medicinal leeches*, in the *J. Reconstr Microsurg, 2004 Aug:20(6); 461-2. The abstract states*, "The medicinal leech, Hirudo Medicinalis, (that is us) has been widely used in the salvage of microvascular free flaps." That is just one of the numerous publications that have detailed the biology, use, b4enefits and risks of leech therapy.

1 Freedman Adam, Clause and Effect. New York Times, Sunday December 18, 2007. Discussion of the Second Amendment's "right to keep and bear arms", emphasizing the importance of the three commas in the Amendment, "A well regulated Militia, being necessary to the security of a free State, and the right of the people to keep and bear Arms, shall not be infringed.

Chapter Eight

William Osler's Mention of Basham's Mixture in the
Treatment of Bright's Disease: Who was Basham and
what was his Mixture?

> Basham's mixture given in plenty of water well
> be found beneficial. (Osler, William, Principles
> and Practices of Medicine, final sentence of
> paragraph   on   Treatment   of   Chronic
> Parenchymatous Nephritis, p. 704, 1892.

The full quotation concerning Basham's mixture under
Treatment of Chronic Parenchymatous Nephritis (large
white kidney with marked dropsy, abundant albumin,
ie: nephrotic syndrome) is quoted   from Osler's text
from 1892 :

> Essentially the same treatment should be carried
> out as in acute Bright's Disease. Milk or
> buttermilk should constitute for a time the chief
> article of food. Later more food may be allowed
> oysters, fresh vegetables, and fruits. The dropsy
> should be treated by the hot baths, and a salt

free diet. Iron preparations should be given when there is marked anaemia. It is to be remembered that the pallor of the face may not be a good index of the blood condition. The acetate of potash, digitalis and diuretin (theobrominae) are useful in increasing the flow of urine. Basham's mixture given in plenty of water will be found beneficial.

Who was Basham and what was the nature of his mixture? This paper will place William Basham in the line of the history of nephrology following Richard Bright's salient paper in 1827, *Reports of Medical Case.* He employed the emerging use of the microscope and the concept of cellular pathology resulting in changes in therapy including the rational for the use of Basham's mixture.

William Richard Basham (1804 – 1877) was born in Diss, a town of 6,700 in north eastern England in Norfolk. It lies in the valley of the River Waveney, around a lake or *mere,* the town taking its name from the Saxon for lake. It is an ancient town, including an early 14th century parish church. It was not until 1831 when he was 27 years old that he enrolled as a student at Westminster Hospital and graduated as a physician a year later from Edinburgh, where Richard Bright and most all English physicians at that time received there medical degrees. Like Bright who took a tour of the continent, Vienna and Hungry before starting practice, Basham made a voyage in the East India Company's ship *Hythe* to China and was wounded in a skirmish. On his return to England it was not until 1843 that he secured the appointment of physician to the Westminter Hospital. Basham became best known for his work on renal diseases., publishing *On Dropsy, and its connection with Diseases of the Kidneys, Heart, Lungs, and Liver* in the year 1858, the year of Richard Bright's death. To quote from Basham's dedication to Richard Bright in this volume:

To Richard Bright, M.D., F.R.S., etc., etc.

Dear Sir: The pathology of the disease which you were the first to describe, and which is inseparable associated with you name, has engaged the attention of many inquirers. The disease has been examined from various points of view, and much as been done to elucidate its causes, its complications, and its progress. The subject however, is not exhausted; and in the following pages I have endeavoured to remove some of the obscurity which still surrounds several points connected with this disease.

It is with sincere and grateful respect that I dedicate these pages to you, animated with the hope that they may assist to place on a true basis the pathology of the disease which bears your name, and contribute to our knowledge of the foretokens of these diseases of the kidney.
I am,
    Dear Sir,
                Very faithfully yours,

                        W.R. Basham

17, Chester Street Grosvenor Place
August 21st, 1858

Bright's recognition of a clinical entity of dropsy and coagulable urine related to renal pathology at autopsy received little recognition initially by his colleagues in London but rather recognition came from Scotland by Robert Christison in his *On Granular Degeneration of the*

Kidnies, in 1839. Christison set the tone of doubt over the significance of the finding, stating that Bright's discoveries *"were received at first with coldness by his brethren. It was said that such cases as he described had been seen only in Guy's Hospital, and in the scum alone of the London population."* In Ireland, Jonathan Osborne (1834) and in France, Pierre Rayer (1839) equally recognized Richard Bright's contributions. But in England it was not until 1858 that William Basham became an equally enthusiastic supporter, *"It is little beyond thirty years since our distinguished countryman, Dr. Bright, laid the foundation by his invaluable and original observations, for a more correct knowledge of these forms of dropsy."*

Like Richard Bright, an accomplished water-color painter, Basham was an excellent draughtsman and many of his illustrations drawn from microscopic appearance of casts in tubules and epithelial lining cells appear in his works. In addition to *On Dropsy*, Basham published a compact volume *Renal Diseases, A Clinical Guide* in 1870, a handbook for the clinician and student. It is in his Croonian Lectures of 1864 on the *Significance of Dropsy* that Basham summaries his approach to dropsy and renal diseases and promulgates his formulation of an iron preparation, thereafter designated as Basham's mixture.

The theme of the first lecture was, "whether our modern methods of investigation *by microscope research are calculated to obtain for us a wider significance for dropsical diseases than has hitherto been accorded to them."* Richard Bright's 1827 *Reports of Medical Cases selected with a View of Illustrating the Symptoms and Cure of Diseases by a Reference to Morbid Anatomy*, was based on gross pathological findings and clinical observation of dropsy and coagulable urine. The unavailability of achromatic microscopic lenses made examination of urine and sections of the kidney not possible. Basham indicated in the first Croonian lecture, *"Bright, however, lived to witness the application of more minute methods of research, and he appreciated highly the results which the microscope was yielding to those who followed in the path he had opened."* Basham had the advantage of being able to use the microscope to study urine and tissue sections, now that achromatic lenses were available and an adequate microtome was available to cut appropriately thin sections of tissue. These factors plus the concept of cellular pathology, advocated by Vichow and others added a new dimension to evaluating underlying disease processes. Basham was to take advantage of these two advances, use of the microscope and importance of cellular patholgy, to look at Bright's Disease in a new way in his text, *On Dropsy,* and summarized in his Croonian lectures.

In this first chapter from the Croonian lectures of 1864, Basham discusses the etiology of dropsy as not being a disease in itself as had previously been considered. He considers three causes of dropsical effusion: 1. "a poor, watery, exhausted blood, a blood deficient in red corpusles, but abounding in white colourless cells (white cells), 2. Presence in the blood of "excrementitious or other noxious material" as might occur in scarlet-fever or with accumulation of urea with impaired renal function, 3. Impediments to the free passage of blood through one or other of the great organ, heart lungs or liver. These naïve causes of dropsy with out demonstrative proof are Basham's alternative to considering dropsy as a disease in itself, as had been considered in the past.

Compare this concept of Dropsy to that of John Elliotson as appears in his 1843 edition of *The Principles and Practice of Medicine* (antedating William Osler's textbook of the same name by forty nine years):

Definition of Dropsy: The next class of affections that we have to consider, belong entirely to serous membranes, and the intestines of the serous cellular tissue. In these cases fluid is secreted in such excess that the ordinary processes of absorption are inadequate for its removal and as the serous cavities of the body are shut sacs, the fluid does not escape, as it does from mucous membranes, so that instead of a discharge or flux, dropsy is the result.

Basham's considers dropsy as more then a condition of the serous membranes but the concept of renal sodium retention as a cause of dropsy would require a more physiological approach to be developed in the future.

Basham then does on to his main thesis that "it is to the very general employment of the microscope in the examination of the excretions during life, as well as of the structure of the organs and tissues after death that we must trace the greater part of the progress that is now being made in the pathology and treatment of these diseases." He credits Virchow and Henle at the University of Berlin stating "that we are chiefly indebted for the extension of the physiology of the cells to the interpretation of the phenomena of disease." While the English lagged behind the European countries in cellular pathology he credits the English school of Mr. Bowman, and Drs. William Addison and Lionel Beale for making advances in this field as well.

Basham gives credit to Dr. Bright who laid the foundations by post-mortem investigation of the significance of the kidneys in the diseases leading to dropsy. However these gross methods of pathology were recognized to have their limits as the microscope provided clues to further information. He continues in this regard, "We find that in every direction in which microscopic research has been hitherto made, evidence has been obtained of alteration in the character of the cellular elements – often times proportioned to, and characteristic of special morbid processes. He recognized that "after Mr. Bowman's description of the basement membrane" or what he calls the germinal membrane is responsible for the succession of single layer of cells forming the renal tubule. "In the early stage of renal disturbance accompanied by albuminous urine and dropsy, the epithelial gland structure of the renal tubes exhibits the simplest and earliest departure from the healthy or physiological type." Plates with drawings by Basham of these changes which are delicate and meticulously drawn accompany the lectures.

Basham puts it succinctly, "The microscope, therefore, as an instrument of investigation should be to the diseases of the kidney, what the stethoscope is to the diseases of the lungs." He discusses changes in the epithelial cells of the tubules with the development of granular and fatty changes and as the disease progresses finally sloughing off in the form of casts that can be examined under the microscope. This would allow an estimate of the progression of the disease process. Basham compares this method of estimating progress of the disease with the then accepted measures, specific gravity or the "weight" of protein or other solids, and finds his use of careful description of the casts under the microscope as equally or perhaps superior to these more established methods.

Continuing along these lines of considering the cell as the basic factor in physiological function as well as pathological changes he states, "It is now universally admitted that the functions of secretion, equally with the process of development and growth, are performed through the agency of the cells...Accordingly we find that in every direction in which microscopic research has been hitherto made, evidence has been obtained of alterations in the character of the cellular elements." He discusses the "healthy" epithelial glands" of the kidney, referring to Mr. Bowman's description of the basement membrane and continues with alterations in "renal disturbance accompanied by albuminous urine and dropsy." He describes and beautifully illustrates changes in epithelial cells in other organs as well. The changes in the composition of the blood, " increase of water and decrease in blood corpuscles" are attributed to these epithelial cell changes. These changes lead to "wide spread decay (in) that the parts and cells which are the seat of it become totally unfit and incapable of ministering to the functions either of nutrition or excretion." He then discussed the origin of "tube-casts in morbus Brightii" quoting the work of George Johnson.

Basham's enthusiastic acceptance of the cellular basis of function and pathology would seem by current standards overdrawn and stretched beyond the limits of the observations. Basham suggests that the albuminuria of chronic renal disease is a secretion related to the abnormalities of the impaired tubular cells. The concept of glomerulo filtration with protein leakage would need to wait consideration for the future.

How Basham's concepts of importance of nutrition and significance of anemia would modify his suggestions for the treatment of chronic renal disease

The importance of supporting the epithelial cells of the renal tubules is used in the second Croonian Lecture to alter the current treatment of chronic renal disease. Basham would eschew the treatment of inflammation, the then current standard goal of therapy, at least in the chronic stage of the disease. Rather than bleeding cupping, and purging, etc as his predecessors would advise, Basham suggested that treatment should be directed "mainly to the renovation of the blood and support and maintenance of its cell forming power." This indeed is a welcome relief from the standard of bleeding, use of leeches, cupping, potassium tartrate and depletions therapies of all sort practiced by the predecessors of Basham, Bright, Christian, Osborne, Rayer, etc. (Bright did not recommend leeches however.)

Consideration of the diet in acute and chronic forms of Bright's disease in this earlier period was hardly recommended and lip service was given to iron therapy or *steel* as it was commonly designated. Diet and iron took on a secondary role to wearing of flannels to avoid chilling, diaphoresis as especially advocated by Osborne, or removal to a warmer or agreeable climate as recommended by Bright, Rayer and even William Osler. Basham substitutes improving the metabolism of cell coupled with correcting the anemia as aims of therapy rather than attack on inflammation. Basham could not free himself however from accepting the then current party line of considering the onset of the disease with its bounding rapid pulse pulse, often fever, and flushed appearance as signs of inflammation, a fire within, needing treatment with depletion therapy, Neither could Basham free himself from the accepted etiology of the condition as related to cold or wet, with alcohol a contributing factor. I t is to be remembered that William Osler accepted these tenants as to etiology and treatment as well.

Basham in reviewing these commonly recommended standards form of treatment rather than dismissing them out of hand, admits they the may be useful in the acute onset of the disease with edema where the features of inflammation may be present. But as the disease progresses attention to the changes in the degenerative changes in the endothelial cells as reflected by examining the urine for casts and the changes in the blood with anemia indicate the need to improved nutrition as well as supplemental iron to correct the anemia and allow the endothelial cells to regenerate. He is firmly against use of bloodletting in this regard.

> Will the abstraction of blood globules from a fluid already exhausted of these, and reduced to a minimum, give aid to renewed cell-growth? In the acute form of the disease I do not affirm that diaphoretics are not needful. I do not affirm that purgatives are not often most salutary in reducing the amount of fluid accumulated in the tissues. I do not say that digitalis is not a most efficient agent in certain stages of these disorders; but I do say that they are each and all insufficient—positively harmful, if not accompanied or followed, according to their action, by agents and remedies intended to fulfill the fundamental principle of treatment, the restoration of the organism of the power of reproduction of those cells which are rapidly disappearing by processes of solution and decay.

> <u>With regard to bloodletting, I unhesitatingly assert that it is injurious: it is manifestly hostile to the fundamental principle on which the treatment of these forms of disease should be based.</u> So long as these disorders were considered as inflammatory, so long as the dropsy was viewed as a product of inflammatory action, such treatment by venesection, or cupping, was only consistent with those doctrines. But here are forms of diseased action in which the blood itself exhibits a deficiency of its most important constituent, in which to take more blood would be but to deteriorate still more the quality of the already impoverished fluid.

Such a strong stand against blood letting at this time was unusual, and seems more emphatic than that of Pierre Louis who in 1825 on statistical basis, *methode numerique,* advocated against bleeding in pneumonia. Even William Osler found bleeding in acute pneumonia a positive benefit and in renal disease something to consider in his text book in 1892. Basham's acceptance of the microscopic findings of cell change and injury in Bright's disease convinced him that nutritional factors affecting the endothelial cells including improving the anemia were of paramount importance.

Basham continues with a more positive approach to the therapy of dropsy with albuminuria, based on recognition of cellular pathological changes as a clue to need for nutritional and supportive modes of therapy.

Rest, warmth, nutritive stimuli, and blood-forming remedies (haematics) are the agents by which this object may be accomplished.

Here Basham turns the tables on the priority for treatment of dropsy. Considering that inflammation was the root cause of the condition Bright, Christian and Rayer, those who established the clinical entity of Bright's disease, all advocated bleeding and depletion therapies to counter act the signs that were considered to indicated inflammation. Osborne in Ireland advocated initially laxatives then diaphoretic measures such as foot, hip or general baths, followed by Dover pills (Ipecac/Opium) as a diaphoretic agent. Lip service was given to what Basham advocated, rest – no one could argue against bed rest to rest the offending organ, warmth – flannels were advocated by Bright and Christison, primarily to prevent chilling, considered an etiological factor in the condition. Nutritive stimuli – "nutritive food of easy digestion and absence of spirituous liquors" was favored by Christison, but not until after blood letting, leeching, depletion measures, counterirritants, laxatives.

Basham's recommendation for the use of blood-forming remedies (haematics) was either ignored or placed low on list of therapeutic measures by the followers of Bright. While describing pallor, Bright doesn't mention use of iron or other agents. Christison who in a footnote described an elegant but laborious method of estimating *hematosin* and anemia as a factor in chronic renal disease as well as after repeated blood letting, follows Bright in ignoring "blood-forming remedies." He did favor the improving nutrition. Rayer after an array of therapeutic agents, teas, laxatives purgative, Sedlitz or Pullna water, etc, recommends that "when the patients are very weak the harsher purgatives are mixed with ferruginous (iron) agents." Robert Elliotson's *Principles and Practices of Medicine* a standard textbook of medicine of 1839 in treating the dropsy of renal disease recommends, "here wine and perhaps good nourishment become necessary, together with steel (iron), sulfate of quinine, and various diuretics."

Basham continues along the same approach he has been advocating. He continues with a list similar to William Osler's conservative approach to management: "Warmth is in itself so essential an element of nutrition that it is only necessary for me to observe here, that a careful attention to maintain the surface of the body at an equable state of temperature by means of flannel clothing, and in the winter time by avoiding an exposure to irregularity of cold are advantages which cannot be over estimated in the management of renal dropsy." Here flannels and the avoidance of cold are justified by their favorable action on nutritive function rather than to prevent relapses of the underlying condition.

Next Basham lists "the influence of pure air, the stimulus given to the blood forming power by the agency of pure air, is too well known to require further remark. In the management of cases in a rank of life where change of residence can be commanded, the sea-side, or resort to localities elevated in situation and possessing the characters of what is called a bracing quality, should be selected." Basham comments more fully in *On Dropsy*, "The influence of pure air, the stimulus given to the blood forming power by the agency of pure air, is too well known to require further remark. In the management of the cases in a rank of life where change of residence can be commanded, the seaside, or resort to localities elevated in situation, and possessing the characters of what is called a bracing quality, should be selected. The influence of sea air in the treatment of chronic albuminuria is most potent, and when the means and circumstances o the patient permit, a sea voyage of some duration should be undertaken. A voyage to Australia offers less variability in the extremes of climate than one to India, and is therefore to be preferred." Osler had recommended removal to Southern California for a similar purpose.

Bashan next takes up "nutritive stimulants." He takes up the "controversial" consideration of whether "alcohol is a nutritive element or not." His predecessors especially Richard Bright listed alcohol as a major cause of the disease. Rather he comes down on the side of Rayer who recommended, "daily use of a ferruginous preparation and a small quantity of good white wine."

I will venture to look at it simply from the clinical point of view without committing myself to the declaration, that wine or alcohol is a nutriment. I will venture, nevertheless, to assert that clinical observation proves it a most efficient (hand-maid) aid to nutritives.---They must be used in moderate quantity, and always in conjunction with food, particularly animal food, either at, or immediately after the meal. They must, on no account, be taken on an empty stomach.--.

It is at this point that Basham begins a discussion of the use of iron and its preparation. "The preparations of iron have long been justly regarded as instrumental in helping to enrich the blood with red corpuscles; and hence appropriately enough called haematemics."

Liquor Ferri et Ammonii Acetatis (Basham's Mixture)

The preparations of iron have long been justly regarded a instrumental in helping to enrich the blood with red corpuscles; and hence appropriately enough called haematics. In all cases where there is evidence of a poor defective blood, called by whatsoever name, anaemia, spanaemia, leukaemia, in the sequel of many acute disease, whether as the result of treatment by bleeding, as was formerly the case in acute rheumatic fever, or from the blood-destroying character of the disease itself, as in the convalescing stage of most fevers, whether continued or intermittent, the rapid and beneficial restorative action of chalybeate medicine or steel (chalybeate and steel implies ferrum or iron) as it is popularly called, particularly in conjunction with animal food and wine, is universally acknowledge and confirmed by daily experience. The preparations of iron in the 'Pharmacopeia' are numerous, but there is one which in these cases of renal dropsy stands pre-eminent for its efficacy and should be preferred in these cases before all others. It is the tincture of the sesquichloride. ($FeCl_3$)

Thus iron in the form of ferric chloride is the basic ingredient of Basham's mixture. Iron was an ancient history and appears in the Ebers Papyrus from Egypt around 1500 BC as a cure for baldness, invoking the suns ray to charm away alopecia and applying a mixture of iron, red-lead, onions, alabaster and honey. The Bible mentions iron many times but not for medicinal purposes. Pierre Blaud in 1832 demonstrated the use of ferrous sulfate combined with potassium carbonate to improve the low iron content of patients with chlorosis (a form of iron deficient anemia). Blaud treated thirty cases of chlorosis in large doses with improvement . Blaud's pills became a staple of the textbooks. Studies in the early twentieth century have shown that ferrous, the reduced form of iron rather than the ferric form is better absorbed from the duodenum, giving some doubt on the superiority of Basham's mixture. But to continue with Basham, since his mixture contains more that just Ferric chloride.

But it is not as the a sesquichloride that its efficacy is most perceived in these cases. It is as an ammonio-chloride, kept in solution by acetic acid, that its beneficial influence becomes most apparent. It is a very simple preparation, a few drops of the tincture (tincture of the sesquichloride, $FeCl3$), according to the age of the patient, are added to a dram of the liquor ammonia acetatis, previously acidulated with acetic acid.

If this is not done-if the sesquichloride is added to the neutral liquor, an insoluble ammonio-chloride falls, which is with difficulty again taken up; but, if the saline is first acidulated a beautiful sherry-red fluid is produced, which is neither unpalatable, nor liable to decomposition and may be kept any time. The tincture of the sesquichloride has long possessed the favorable opinion of physicians in most cases of renal or genito-vesical disorder.

It is this last paragraph that deserves the most attention. Could it have been that it was that *beautiful sherry-red fluid* that most attracted Basham to his mixture ? The fact that the preparation was soluble and not liable to precipitation, as Blaud's pills were, and that the mixture was *neither unpalatable, nor liable to decomposition and may be kept any time* all add to its advantage. It is to be noted that opinions differ as to its stability and the U.S. Dispensatory 24 edition of 1947 has some reservations in this regard. But it is this last statement of Basham, *The tincture of the sesquichlorid has long possessed the favorable opinion of physicians in most cases of renal or genito-vesical disorder* that is most problematic. No case studies are reported to testify to the effectiveness of this mixture, as was the case with Blaud pills where 30 cases were reported in 1832 on their effectiveness in chlorosis. The U.P. Dispensatory comments on this point as well denying Basham's claim for the mixture, Basham's statement to the contrary. William Olser recommended iron in various preparations in his text book (perchloride, ie: $FeCl3$ alone, $FeI3$, $Fe(PO4)3$ other than as Basham's mixture). I wonder if Osler's recommendation for the use of Basham's mixture which only appears in this chapter on Bright's disease may not have been based on its role as an hematemic, but rather stemming on general principles from the authority of Basham's statement in this Croonian lecture.

Let us again look at Osler's paragraph which mentions Basham's mixture in the very last sentence of the paragraph. Use of iron preparations, without particular choice noted, for anemia is already mentioned several lines above. Basham's mixture is like a parting gesture, a casual throw away thought, a wave to authority. Was Osler equally infatuated with the color, that beautiful sherry red color or was it as noted by Basham that "the tincture of the sesquichloride has long possessed the favorable opinion of physicians ?" Hot baths, acetate of potash, digitalis and a diuretic often a mercurial but with Osler a milder theobromine preparation, were commonly used by Bright and his followers. Osler's recommendation of a low salt diet in contrast was a relatively recent concept in the treatment of dropsy, not to be found in the writings of the nascent nephrologists from Bright to Basham earlier in the century.

Indeed the anemia of chronic renal disease is not primarily an iron deficient anemia but it wasn't until 1957 that a hormone produced in the kidney, Erythropoietin, was shown by Jacobson to be the main factor in the anemia of chronic renal disease. (Hemolysis and blood loss are minor factors in the anemia of renal disease. I remember performing chromium tagged red blood cells studies for Dr. C.V.Moore in St. Louis in the early 1950ies demonstrating a mild hemolytic component.) The effectiveness of Erythropoietin has been overwhelmingly demonstrated in the chronic dialysis population, significantly raising the hematocrit. Iron alone is ineffective but in combination with Erythropoietin considerably improves the quality of life of patients with chronic renal failure. Basham as well as William Osler I am sure would have welcomed these results as an improvement on Basham's Mixture.

Summary:

Basham acknowledged his indebtedness to Richard Bright for recognizing the relationship between dropsy, coagualable urine and renal disease. He was able to employ the microscope and the concept of cellular pathology to consider more carefully the significance of the tube casts and their possible significance in the understanding of renal disease. Basham, while not able to throw off the concept of inflammation as the initial pathological factor in initiation of renal disease, used his concept of the importance of nutrition and the quality of the blood in the chronic phase to condemn bleeding and other efforts at depletion therapy directed towards inflammation. He recommended an iron preparation, *Liquor Ferri et Ammonii Acetatis* (Basham's Mixture) that remained in the pharmological texts for over one hundred years and made it into William Osler's text as one of the agents in the treatment of renal disease.

Chapter Nine

Sir William Osler's View on Pierre C.A. Louis'
Recommendations for Bleeding In Pneumonia—
Paradox of Calling his Method Iconoclastic
Continuing Practice of Bleeding

"La Barriere contre l'esprit du systeme"

"Medicina est ars conjecturalis"

"There are many stars in Paris, but Louis is the sun"

Objectives

1. Review of background leading to Pierre Louis'questioning of bleeding in pneumonia

2. Evaluate Louis' *methode numerique* with emphasis on careful observation and enumeration of results

3. Explain William Osler's admiration of Pierre Louis, including his Essay on *The Influence of Louis on American Medicine* and visiting his tomb, yet his continuing recommendations for bleeding in pneumonia in spite of Louis' studies showing the "narrow limits to the utility of this mode of treatment."

In the third edition of William Osler's Principles and Practice of Medicine, 1897, regarding recommendations for bleeding in pneumonia, are the lines:

> The reproach of van Helmont that a bloody Molock presides in the chairs of medicine cannot be brought against the present generation of physicians.

Before Louis' iconoclastic paper on bleeding in pneumonia it would have been considered almost criminal to treat a case without venesection.

During the first five decades of the century the profession bled too much, but during the last decade we have certainly bled too little. Pneumonia is one of the diseases in which a timely venesection may save lives. To be of service it should be done early"

Pierre Louis' paper, *Researches on the Effect of Bloodletting in some Inflammatory Disease*, published in 1828 called into question the value of phlebotomy in pneumonia. How then could William Osler call Louis' paper iconoclastic and in the same breath recommend that bleeding should be performed more frequently and early as well? Textbooks contemporaneous with Osler's *Principles and Practice of Medicine* by Alfred Loomis and Austin Flint had found little to recommend bleeding in pneumonia at the end of the 19th century. Oliver Wendell Holmes in his farewell address at the Harvard Medical

School in 1882 referred to bloodletting as a past "wonder-worker in disease now thankfully discarded."

William Olser was an admirer of Pierre Louis and praised him in the essay on *The Influence of Louis on American Medicine* as well as visiting his grave in Paris in 1905. Osler in this paper on Louis quotes correctly Louis's conclusions, 1. "pneumonia is never arrested at once by blood letting" and 2. "the supposed happy effects on the progress of the disease were very much less than was commonly believed." Recognizing these conclusions why did Osler not follow Louis' advice and temper his use of blood letting in pneumonia? Why the enthusiasm of Osler for bleeding in pneumonia? Did Osler have an alternative interpretation of the results of Louis, or did he consider that the data were not entirely convincing? Could there have been other reasons for his position which was against the grain of prevailing medical opinion at the time? These are the questions to be considered in this paper.

Louis' Method

Louis' method was to gather together a sufficient number of cases of a similar condition and tabulate them so that the results of therapeutic maneuver could be evaluated. He stressed the importance of accurate observation, carefully describing the historical and clinical condition to be as certain as possible that the subjects all had a similar condition. He divided the patients into a group treated early and a group with similar diagnostic features treated later in the disease, noting time of onset and convalescence. Perhaps is was this empirical method and its careful execution that Osler could have considered *iconoclastic* in his paper rather than the interpretation or conclusion of the results.

Louis could find little difference between the effectiveness of early or late bleeding.

Osler in his essay on Louis, rather than focusing on Louis' methods and conclusions placed great emphasis on the influence of Louis on the many young American physicians such as James Jackson, Jr., Henry I. Bowditch, Oliver Wendell Holmes etc, who went to Paris in the 1830's and brought back with them an approach to medicine mirroring that of their teacher. It was these Americans and other foreign students who studied with Louis who organized the Society of Medical Observation (*Mediale d'Observation*) where frequent debates on theory and practice of medicine took place. Let us briefly review some of these debates as they set the stage for evaluating Louis' methods.

Debate at the Royal Academy of Medicine in Paris

An example of such a debate at the Royal Academy of Medicine in Paris was between M. Francois Double who argued for the "Inapplicability of Statistics to the Practice of Medicine" and Pierre Louis who supported the Application of Statistics to Medicine. These debates translated into English with editorial comments were published in the *American Journal of the Medical Sciences* in 1837, very soon after the original debates took place. The editors of this journal for the most part had been students of Louis and were anxious to place before American medicine insight into these current proceedings and other developments in French medicine.

M. Francois Double was a practitioner of the old school, favoring the authority of the ancients and supporting the physician's ability to modify therapy based on the individual characteristics of his patient rather than an *arithmetical* mean obtained from the juggling of numbers.

At the time there was considerable controversy over whether mathematical treatment of clinical information was appropriate."

Let M. Double speak for the large group of skeptics with a quotations from his arguments in this debate:

> The science of statistics is in these days one of the most fashionable; and in the ardor of their zeal its disciples have applied it indiscriminately to medicine....If (it) ever be effected, medicine would cease to be either a science, an art or even a profession: <u>it would become as mechanical as the employment of the shoemaker.</u>

M. Double continues with one of his major points, "Each of our problems embraces but one individual and besides, diseases always have their prevailing character, varying progressively according to an infinite variety of causes."

And how would Pierre Louis answer this blistering attack of M. Double on the duty of the practitioner to respect the individual variation in patients and the weight of past medical practice, tempered with his own knowledge and experience?

Pierre Louis begins his argument with a straight forward declaration, "A therapeutic agent cannot be employed with any discrimination or probability of success in a given case, unless its general efficacy in analogous cases has been previously ascertained:

> "therefore I conceive that without the aid of statistics nothing like real medical science is possible." In conclusion, Louis states, "the numerical analysis which is of no use without

numerous and well observed facts, must in turn have a great influence in rendering perfect the observation of fact."

Such debates revolved around whether clinical medicine was an art dealing with the individual patient as suggested by Double or required an empirical approach with groups of patients, as suggested by Louis. If William Osler had been at these debates is it possible he would have sided more with Double in the importance of the individual patient against numerical results from groups of patients?

Louis' study on bleeding in pneumonia did not have a comparison group of non-treatment patients that would have made his conclusions more compelling, but considering the weight of authority that bleeding had in inflammatory conditions at that time it probably would have been impossible to have had such a controlled group. Ironically von Helmont's text of 1649 which William Osler conjured up with reference to *"a bloody Molock presides in the chairs of medicine,"* had suggested such a prospective clinical trial. Von Helmont was opposed to bleeding himself primarily on basis of religious argument that the blood was the site of the soul. Pierre Louis as well described a hypothetical study involving two comparable groups of patients, as in an epidemic, arbitrarily treating one group with one form of therapy and the other with a different mode and comparing the results. Neither of these suggested studies were ever carried out however. A controlled therapeutic trial was carried out on May 1747 by the Scotchman James Lind aboard the *Salisbury* to evaluate treatment of scurvy with unequivocal results using two oranges and one lemon.

Let us consider some background of the medical career of Pierre Louis and how it was a factor leading to his questioning of the value of blood letting in pneumonia.

Pierre Charles Alexandre Louis (1787 – 1872)
Background

The Paris school of medicine prepared Louis for his studies on treatment of pneumonia as well as his work on tuberculosis, yellow fever and typhoid fever. Louis came rather late to his role as a clinical scientist, having spent several years in Russia as a clinician following graduation from medical school. He became troubled by the meager medical knowledge available to manage children with diphtheria and returned to France determined to spend the next seven years just observing and evaluating the course and treatment of a variety of illnesses.

He was helped in this endeavor by his contemporaries Andral and Chomel who provided him space in the hospitals to evaluate the clinical course and treatment of a number of conditions.

Louis' Studies with Bloodletting in Pneumonia

Louis originally published his observation on the treatment of pneumonia as *Memoires et Observations* in 1828 where 78 patients at the hospital *la Pitie* were studied. This is the opening page of the *Memoires* with a table of results where are tabulated 50 of the patients that survived, 28 were fatal and discussed later. More legible is the table from the expanded publication of 1835, *Researches on the Effect of Bleeding in Some Inflammatory Diseases*, translated into English in the following year by C.G. Putnam with additional studies by James Jackson. The figures on the horizontal line above the columns indicate the day bleeding began after onset. The figures to the left in each column mark the duration of the disease, as defined by Louis, those to the right the number of bleedings, and those on the horizontal line below show on the left the mean duration of the disease and to the right the average number of bleedings.

Louis grouped together those bleed during the first two days of illness as representing *early bloodletting* (6 patients) and the remaining 44 patients bleed later in their course, third through the ninth day, *late bloodletting*. The length of the illness in these very few patients (6) who were bled early averaged eleven days, much shorter than the mean of 20.3 day for those bleed later.

This reduced length of illness may have been a factor leading to William Olser's recommendation for bleeding early in pneumonia. Remember Osler dictum, "To be of service bleeding should be done early."

However Louis is very quick to comment on this finding, recognizing that the sample size was too small and if more cases had been examined these differences "would have been considerably less."

In addition he considered that those admitted later in the course of the illness had "committed errors of regimen, strong drink and brandy, resulting in increase in the length of the disease", making the average length of illness of those bleed late, 20.3 days, falsely long.

Louis then resorts to an alternative interpretation of the data, "so that we should get nearer the truth "—by taking the mean duration of the disease in cases bled during the four first days: and on the other (hand) in those who were not bled until the fifth to the ninth inclusive. Then the mean duration of pneumonitis would be seventeen days among the first group, bleed early and twenty days among the second group bleed later." Louis has changed the definition of early from the first two days to the first four days, because the number of subjects from days one and two were small. The difference between bleeding early and late with this alternative definition of early bleeding leads to a less striking difference, average duration by new definition, 17 days as compared to later, 20 days for those bleed later.

Louis' efforts to Insure Comparability of the Group of Patients

Louis was very careful to indicate that the groups were comparable, that the "violence of the disease" and character of treatment was "equally energetic and directed by the same physician." He also was careful to note that the severity of the disease was comparable in the two groups, considering the physical findings in the chest such as "crepitation, resonance of voice, egophony, dullness on percussion as well as acceleration of pulse, 'heats' and sweats." He judged the onset of disease as the onset of fever and appearance of "pain on one side of the chest and rusty sputum; and I have regarded as the time of convalescence the period at which the sick began to take some light nourishment, three days at least after the febrile action had ceased.

Louis discusses the progression of each of these particular symptoms and signs and found little alteration following bleeding. He concludes, "that the utility of bleeding has been very limited in the cases thus far analyzed."

Fatal Cases

Louis next discusses the 28 fatal cases. Remember William Osler dictum "Pneumonia is one of the diseases in which a timely venesection may save lives" which does not seem to be well supported by the following results.

Of the patients bleed in the first four day, the alternative definition of early the early group, 18 died out of a total of 41 or 3/7 (43 %), while whose bleed later, after the 4th day, nine died of the 36 or only one quarter (25%).

Louis considered that this higher mortality in the early treated group was related to age of patients, the earlier treated group had a mean age was 41 and that of the later group 38.

Louis concludes, "Thus the study of the general and local symptoms, the mortality and variations in the mean duration of the pneumonitis, according to the period at which bloodletting was instituted; all establish narrow limits to the utility of this mode of treatment."

And then as a final point, Louis considers sarcastically the questions, "Should we obtain more important (more favorable) results if, as is practiced in England, the first bleeding were carried to syncope?" Marshall Hall in England to whom Louis had dedicated his Researches, had recommended near syncope as a guide to dosing bleeding in various conditions.

Use of Statistics in Louis' Data

Louis' paper evaluated a procedure considered sacred from the time of Hippocrates, sitting abreast a most enthusiastic period for massive bleeding and leeching as proposed by Broussaais at that time for almost every medical condition. Considering the climate of the times he was remarkable for his audacity to question bleeding in an inflammatory disease.

Louis, however recognized that the relative small number of patients treated limited the significance of his conclusions. In addition there were no control groups, only averages and means.

This was not because the French didn't have the basic background in such mathematical studies.

French mathematicians such as Laplace, Fournier, and Poisson had applied theory of probability to gaming, astronomical, mortality and population studies.

As a physician dedicated to careful collection and organization of clinical data Louis can perhaps be excused for not applying the then known mathematical theory to medical data where it had never been applied before.

Jules Gavarret a physician with mathematical training had applied probability calculations to Louis' mortality data to his studies in typhoid fever and indicated a lack of validity because of the limited number of observations.

As pointed out by Alvan R. Feinstein, "As a pioneer in clinical statistics, Louis helped end the popularity of blood-letting by counting and comparing the results of patients treated in various ways. His general statistical techniques had many defects...only with the advent of antibiotics to treat infectious disease, medical statistics finally reached the era of the therapeutic clinical trial." This was however over 100 years after Louis' original observations.

Possible Explanations for Osler's Continued
Recommendations for Bleeding in Pneumonia

The task remains to reconcile Osler's acknowledgement
and praise of Pierre Louis' *methode numerique* with faint
damming of his recommendations for bleeding in
pneumonia. Let us consider several possible
explanations for Osler's justification for early bleeding in
pneumonia.

He could have invoked Gavarret's 1840 criticism of the
validity of Louis' data where statistical theory is applied,
but there is no indication that Olser was acquainted with
this criticism.

Or perhaps Osler's focus on the individual patient,
physician's experience and judgment as emphasized by
Double in the debates may have tempered his
acceptance of numerical data obtained from groups of
patients?

Alternately Osler might have seen in pneumonia a
component of heart failure indicating bleeding. He lists
in his text book other conditions not only heart failure
but cerebral hemorrhage and hypertension, or increased
"arterial tension" as he called it, where bleeding is
recommended. Until potent diuretics were developed
bleeding was an accepted treatment of severe heart
failure. A recent unpublished paper by our chairman,
 Dr. Charles S. Bryan et al, *Bloodletting for Pneumonia:
Closure to a Controversy*, reviewed the data that supports
the findings that perhaps one quarter of patients with
pneumonia may have evidence of heart failure.

Or did William Osler's emphasis on Louis' contribution
and influence on training a group of physicians who
created an American school of clinical medicine trump

the importance of the results of the *methode numerique* in initiating the demise of bleeding in pneumonia?

Osler and subsequent editors continued to recommend bleeding in pneumonia throughout subsequent editions of the *Principles and Practice of Medicine* through 1944.

Major Greenwood has considered that, "Louis indeed seemed more honoured in America than France and Osler honoured him not so much as the inventor of the numerical method as the teacher of the Americans such as James Jackson, Bowditch, Oliver Wendell Homes and William Gerhard." This appraisal is somewhat confirmed by Arnold C. Klebs who accompanied Osler to Louis' mausoleum at the Montparnasse Cemetery in 1905 recalling Osler's actual remarks, "Louis has a far higher claim on our affection and gratitude, as through his students he may have be said to have created the American school of clinical medicine." Such was Olser's assessment of Louis and as for his results in his *Researches on the Effect of Bloodletting in Pneumonia*, they are not mentioned at the tomb that day.

At the time of the American's visit to Louis' tomb, Pierre Louis' reputation had fallen to such a low points that according to Cushing in his biography of Osler, "no one, not even the French physicians who were consulted, had any idea where Louis was buried." Cushing added to Osler's remarks as remembered by Klebs at the tomb, noting "the sad death of his son at the age of eighteen from tuberculosis, of his [Louis'] own death from the same disease at the age of eighty—five; of his special claims to remembrance—not so much his attempt to introduce mathematical accuracy into the study of disease, [but] his higher claim to have created the American school of clinical medicine through his pupils." Erwin Ackerknecht summarized Louis' bitter sweet later life, "He was condemned to live to a very advanced age, and to be the sad survivor of his young son, his dearest pupils such as Jackson, his closest friends like Chomel and Marshall Hall, and of his own importance.

Summary

1. Background on Pierre Louis' studies on bleeding in pneumonia showing "narrow limits to the utility of this mode of treatment."

2. Debates at the Royal Academy of Medicine on the applicability of statistics to medicine

3. Evaluation of Louis's results in treating 78 patients with pneumonia with bloodletting

4. Lack of statistical methods applied by Louis to his studies in spit of French mathematician's studies in gaming, astronomy and mortality tables.

5. Discussion of reasons for William Osler's continued recommendations for bleeding in pneumonia in spite of his labeling Louis' method *iconoclastic,* writing an essay on his contributions to American medicine and visiting his grave in 1905.

Systeme de Broussais Broussais instructs a nurse to extract even more blood from a pallid patient with leeches on his chest and blood dripping from all over his body.

Patient: "But I have no more than a drop of blood in my veins."

Btousseau " Never mind, 50 more leeches."

Chapter Ten

Sir William Osler—A Departure from his Reputation as a Therapeutic Conservative—The Treatment of   Bright's Disease

A desire to take medicine is, perhaps, the great feature which distinguishes people from other animals.   William Osler   Science, 17, 170, 1891

Summary

Sir William Osler's textbook, *The Principles and Practice of Medicine*, first edition 1892 addressing treatment of acute and chronic Bright's Disease contains many echoes of antiphlogistic treatments including depletion therapy of the earlier nineteenth century.   Procedures recommended by Osler include bleeding, and other depletion therapies, mercurial diuretics in the form of Calomel, laxatives such as Jalap and Cream of Tartar, application of the cautery to the loins and cupping, as well as warm baths, Pilocarpine, and the use of Canton flannels to encourage sweating. All these therapeutic measures were recommended by Richard Bright and his followers, Robert Christison, Jonathan Osborne and Pierre Rayer earlier in the century. Such procedures are strikingly absent in Osler's consideration of other diseases, such as Tuberculosis and Typhoid fever, where he is more in compliance with his reputation as a conservative therapeutic nihilist. The recommendations for treatment of Renal Disease by Bright and his followers, Christison, Osborne, and Rayer in the early nineteenth century will be compared with what appears in the initial and subsequent editions of Osler's text.

Introduction

William Osler in addition to his many accolades, as a kind compassionate physician with an encyclopedic knowledge of literature and author of *The Principles and Practice of Medicine*, first edition 1892, was considered a therapeutic conservative, reducing and eliminating outmoded and archaic forms of management, favoring supportive care, diet and non aggressive approach to the treatment of medical conditions. His discussion of the treatment and management of Typhoid Fever in the first chapter of his Text is an excellent example of such an approach: "The profession was long in learning that typhoid is not a disease to be treated mainly with drugs. Careful nursing and a regulated diet are the essentials in a majority of the cases."[1] He goes on to detail the need for a well-ventilated room, the characteristics of the bed for comfort and convenience of care, and above all, "an intelligent nurse should be in charge." Typhoid mouth wash (carbolic acid 4 c. cc, glycerine 30 c.c., saturated solution of boric acid to 300c.c.) was still on the Hospital Formulary in 1950 when I was a student on the wards. In considering therapeutic measures Osler most often was frank to admit that no specific treatment was indicated and above all to avoid harmful measures. Following this he often recommended general supportive measures such as diet, details of nursing and general supportive care and in the case of Typhoid fever details on how the stools should be collected. Then would follow measures often steeped in tradition, often more vigorous treatments that could be considered on a take it or leave it basis, but seemed to be less recommended. Indeed Osler's sections on therapy were initially considered the weakest part of the Text. Style, historical perspective, a diseased based catalogue of illness based on pathological data were all considered the stronger points in the Text. Frederick T. Gates, a confidant of John D. Rockefeller having read the book, was so struck by the absence of specific therapeutic measures that could lead to a cure, that he recommended to Rockefeller an institute that could address these need. The ambiguity of the therapeutic sections of The Principles and Practice of Medicine in this led to the establishment of the Rockerfeller Institutue of Medical Research.

An examination of the sections on the treatment of Acute and Chronic Bright's Disease however, will show however that while his conservative approach was maintained, he followed many of the suggested treatments and procedures of those of sixty-five years earlier when Bright originally published his *Reports on Medical Cases* in 1827. These included procedures and practices as well from the physicians who closely followed and confirmed Bright's findings, Robert Christison in Scotland, Jonathan Osborne from Ireland, and Pierre Rayer in Paris, France. Osler's discussion of the treatment and management of renal disease demonstrates many similarities and a tacit acceptance of these older and more aggressive modes of therapy. Is it believable that Sir William would endorse mercury in the form of calomel, strophanthus, strychnia, digitalis, bleeding, cupping, saline laxatives as well as jalap, Elaterium and Cream of Tartar (Potassium Bitartrate), application of the cautery to the loins, warm baths, and pilocarpine to induce sweating? It is true Osler's section on the treatment of Bright's disease doesn't include potent laxatives such as Scammony (root from Asia Minor and Syria), and Gamboge (gum resin from E. Indian tree) as did his earlier colleagues from the first part of the century. Nor does Osler mention use of leeches, cantharides (a genius of beetles or Spanish fly) or Dover pills (Ipecac and Opium). However, as Osler's text is reviewed with reference to the use of prior therapeutic armamentaria from the physicians who established the clinical entity of Bright's Disease, coagulable urine, dropsy, and granular kidneys, a striking similarity and congruence will be apparent.

In addition to the general measures of treatment of renal disease, diet, bed rest, and keeping the patient warm, William Osler advocated efforts to promote sweating, warm poultices, hydrotherapy, guarding against the cold or change of climate, and residence to a "warm, equable climate." These were all measures having their origin in consideration of the general theory of disease of the early nineteenth century going back to Galen. These were part of the antiphlogistic theory of disease where bleeding and loss of fluids from the bowel and skin were considered to redress the hyperdynamic circulation and other components of inflammation (from *inflammare*–to set on fire). The skin was considered as an organ in the modulation of disease by its ability to breathe and open pores to eliminate noxious products. In addition there was the general notion of a sympathetic alliance between bowel, skin and kidney that needed to be brought back into harmony to promote health. The early nineteenth century also employed depletion therapy in the form of bleeding and laxatives to combat "inflammation," a loosely conceived concept that included fever often supported by a buffy coat appearance of the extracted blood. Bright early on recognized the presence of dropsy or edema accompanied at times by pleural effusions, cardiac involvement, and central nervous system signs. He labeled these "inflammatory affections" (*affection* — commonly used in the early nineteenth century to indicated a disease or morbid condition, rather than a warm tender feeling) and it was toward these manifestations that therapy was directed.

William Osler's 1892 edition of *Principles and Practice* as well as later editions will be examined to see if he presented a through-going conservative approach, a rigorous cleansing of these older principles from the earlier part of the century, or whether echoes of the older therapeutic principles come through.

Examination of Osler's Text: Principles and Practice of Medicine (1892)
Bed Rest

Osler's first edition of The Principles and Practice of Medicine of 1892, begins by stating that in the treatment of Acute Bright's Disease: "The patient should be in bed and there remain until all tracers of the disease have disappeared." Jonathan Osborne, a physician in Dublin Ireland who confirmed Bright's work adding observations of his own in his 1833 publication On the nature and treatment of dropsical diseases states, "When a patient is placed under my care with generalized edema, coaguable urine and dry skin, the first thing is to keep him in bed to maintain warmth of surfaces." Osborne was convinced that suppression of sweating was the cause of the disease and recommended many measures to induce sweating, warm baths, emersion of extremities in water, or vapour baths, foot baths, hip baths etc. Leading directly to Osler's next sentence:" As sweating plays such an important part in the treatment, it is well, if possible to accustom the patient to blankets. He should be clad in thin Canton flannel." (Canton flannel according to the Fabric Catalog is a cloth originally made in Canton, China, being a strong and absorbent cotton cloth made with a basic common twill weave using a soft, loosely spun weft). However Osler was not the first to recommend flannels. Richard Bright in his Cases and Observations of 1836, states, "With a view to keeping up the action of the skin, I have been very careful in pointing out to those who have not been confined by the disease, the necessity of wearing an inner dress of flannel at all times." Pierre Rayer in his Traite des Maladies des Reins et des Alterations de la Secretion Urinaire (Treatise on Diseases of the Kidneys and Alterations of Urinary Secretion) states, "...and one should take care to keep the body warm by suitable clothing. If the weather is cold, even though the apartment might be well heated, one of the best ways of preventing a relapse is by covering the body with flannel." John Osborne was also an advocate of flannels, "Individuals who have been relieved from dropsy by restoration of the function of the skin, are liable to relapse if exposed to cold, so as to produce return of the cutaneous obstruction. Hence they ought to wear flannel next the skin and to make a timely use of bathes and frictions in care of dryness of the surface recurring." Yet another champion of flannels for their affect in augmenting sweating and contributing to the skin's function in compliance of the depletion theory of disease was Robert Christison. He was an early champion of Richard Bright's concept of renal disease and stated, "The body should be warmly clothed, protected against sudden exposure to cold, especially cold and wet together. A general flannel dress should be constantly worn." Osler seems to have accepted the underlying premise of the earlier 19th Century that the skin as an organ needed to be relieved of its obstruction to promote health. The ubiquitous use of flannels is also apparent.

Diet

Returning to Osler: "The diet should consist of milk or butter milk, gruels made of arrow-root or oat-meal, barley water and, if necessary beef tea and chicken broth. It is better, if possible, to confine the patient to a strictly milk diet." Osler justified his use of milk in the section on Typhoid fever, indicating that " milk is digested with great ease, leaving behind the smallest amout of residue to form feces" Rayer also recommended milk stating that the diet should be that of an acute inflammatory disease. "*I have seen patients do well with nothing but* milk *as food for a few days.*" In the section on Chronic Bright's Disease, Osler cautions, "The patient should be warned not to eat meat more than once a day." Here Osler takes a conservative approach to treatment, emphasizing the Greek practice of the importance of diet. This attention to diet is often missing in the treatment program of Bright and his followers. Rayer in the treatment of Case 8, a young man of 16 years old, living on a very damp ground floor presenting with anasarca and coaguable urine, recommended steam baths and tapping of first the right and then the left chest (fluid had been detected by "taping and listening to the chest"), followed by leeches, vesicatories, and high doses of calomel, etc. Osler's therapeutic conservatism is in striking contrast to Rayer in this regard and only as an after-thought, did Rayer recommend "*a bland diet with* milk."   The concept of reducing protein in the diet, to decrease nitrogen and urea production, as well as restriction of salt were unknown to the original nephrologists. Osler's recommendation to restrict meat, but paradoxically to recommend a high source of protein in milk is somewhat of a contradiction. Not until the seventh and last edition of *The Principles and Practice of Medicine* of 1909 that was solely edited by William Osler, was the importance of salt restriction finally recognized, "As there is marked retention of chlorides, which seem to bear a relation to the dropsy, salt should be with held." Bright and his followers, Christison, Osborne, and

Rayer, gave no consideration to salt as a factor in the development of edema and ascites.

Cream of Tartar

The third paragraph of Osler's treatment of acute Bright's Disease: "The patient should drink freely of alkaline mineral waters, ordinary water, or lemonade. The fluids keep the kidneys flushed and wash out the debris from the tubes. A useful drink is a drachm (4 ml) of <u>cream of tartar</u> in a pint of boiling water, to which may be added the juice of a half of lemon and a little sugar. Bright also was especially enthusiastic about the use of <u>Cream of Tarter</u> or the Supertartrate of Potash (a diuretic and cathartic). To quote from his section on Observations on the Treatment from Reports of Medical Cases Selected with a view of Illustration the Symptoms and Cure of Diseases by a Reference to Morbid Anatomy: "Purgatives generally act well; the Elaterium in the case of Case XIV, Leonard Evans evidently gave much relief; and all the saline laxatives which unite a certain degree of diuretic power are decidedly useful. Amongst these I have found the <u>Supertartrate of Potash</u> the most efficacious; and the best mode of exhibiting it when the stomach will admit, is by directing the patient to take a large draught of a mixture containing more of the salt than the water will dissolve, the first thing in the morning: and it will be seen that in some cases I have almost trusted entirely to the remedy. Where the stomach will not bear this mode of administering purgatives, the combination of Jalap, <u>Supertertartrate of Potash</u> and a little Ginger repeated from time to time, answers well." Osler didn't mention the Jalap and substituted "half a lemon and a little sugar" for Bright's "little Ginger" On the other hand Rayer in a long footnote in the Traite indicates his displeasure with Dr. Christison who, "brags especially about the effects of combined action of <u>cream of tarter</u> and digitalis—After three of four days of the simultaneous use of these two remedies, Dr. Christison says the diuresis is established. This diuresis is sometimes influenced by the administration of a mercury pill each evening for four or five days. When these diuretics have been taken for some time, Dr. Christison continues, 'I have sometimes seen their action take hold suddenly, after the administration of an <u>emetic of tartar (antimony potassium tartrate)</u> impregnated with antimony of ipecac, and often after a single dose of a hydragogous cathartic (one that produces a watery discharge), such as gamboges." Rayer by his introduction, " Dr. Christison brags" seems to indicate his incredulity over Christison's results. Certainly Osler didn't add mercury, ipecac or gambage to his cream of tarter.

Cupping, Cautery, Poultice

Osler shows his more conservative and cautious role in the first part of the next paragraph, but then regresses to the earlier party line on the relationship of the bowel, skin, and kidneys:" No remedies, so far as known, control directly the changes which are going on in the kidneys. The indications (for remedies) are: 1. To give the excretory function of the kidney rest by utilizing the skin and bowels, in hope that the natural processes may be sufficient to effect a cure, 2. to meet the symptoms as they arise." Up to this point Osler demonstrates a through going conservative approach.

Osler continues with therapeutic recommendation more in line with physicians of the earlier part of the century in the second part of this sixth paragraph on the treatment of renal disease in the 1892 edition of *The Principles and Practices of Medicine*, "At the onset when there is pain in the back or haematuria, the dry or wet cups give relief. The last should not be used in children. Warm poultices are often grateful. In cases which set in with suppression of urine these measures are adopted, and in addition the hot bath with subsequent pack, copious diluents, and a free purge." Richard Bright, Osborne, Christison, and especially P. Rayer all advocated cupping. Cupping was a procedure developed in China and used in Eastern Europe, where metal or glass cups, often warmed, were applied to the skin and the suction allegedly stimulated the underlying circulation. Wet cupping consisted of making an incision in the skin and then applying a cup to extract blood. Richard Bright reported that William Brooks, Case XVIII on December 20, 1816 was, *"a good deal relieved by cupping."* Rayer reported in *Traite des Maladies des Reins*, *"among the successful remedies, one must put in first place, general blood letting and the application of cupping glasses in the lumbar region. In individuals of strong constitution, the amount of blood to be let should be in proportion to the rise in temperature and to the rapidity with which the dropsy has developed. With children, in the first application of the cupping glasses, ordinarily about 4-6 ounces of blood are extracted; in an adult 8-10 ounces."* While Rayer may recommend a smaller volume of blood to be removed in cupping of children, Osler's admonishes not to use wet cupping at all. Osler is rather vague on the nature of "warm poultices", Bright is more specific in recommending to his first and famous patient, John King on the 31st of October, 1825, *Applicetur emplast Cantharides Sterno* (application of a poultices of cantharidis, ie: dried Spanish Fly or Blister bug, to the sternum).

Baths and Stimulation of the Skin with Pilocarpine

To continue with Sir William: "In cases which set in with suppression of urine these measures (dry and wet cups) should be adopted, and in addition the dropsy is best treated by hydrotherapy—either the hot bath, the wet pack or the hot-air bath. In children the wet pack is usually satisfactory. It is applied by wringing a blanket out of hot water, wrapping the child in it, covering this with a dry blanket and then with a rubber cloth. In the case of adults, the hot air bath or the vapor bath may be conveniently given by allowing the vapor or air to pass from a funnel beneath the bed clothes, which are raised on a low cradle; sweating produced by these measures is usually profuse, rarely exhausting, and in a majority of cases the dropsy can in this way be relieved. There are some cases, however, in which the skin does not respond to the baths, and if the symptoms are serious, particularly if uraemia supervenes, Jaborandi or its active principle, pilocarpine, may be used."

Warm baths and wet packs to produce sweating were a common recommendation of Osborne, Christison and Rayer. Jonathan Osborne considered the etiology of the disease to be "Anhidrosis" and recommended vigorous use of "foot, hip and general baths or vapor baths to be given an hour before bed." P. Rayer is an even more champion of baths: "In our Hospital, as in common practice, it is necessary to give baths near the bed of the patient so that he does not get cold in the trip from the bath to his bed. In cold weather especially, patients should never be transported to the bathroom. When the baths are taken in convalescence by people who have been getting up already for a few days, it is preferable to give the baths in the evening, shortly before the patient goes to sleep." Rayer continues, "When gastric or intestinal symptoms, and in particularly if vomiting and diarrhea are very pronounced, warm baths, leeches on the anus, and small doses of opium are salutary remedies." Osler agreed with Rayer's warm baths and small doses of opium but eschewed the use of leeches.

Laxatives and Other Depletion Therapies: Jalop, Elaterium, and Bleeding

Osler continues and all of his earlier colleagues agree: "The bowels should be kept open by a morning saline purge. The compound powder of jalap or if necessary, elaterium may be used. If these measures fail to reduce the dropsy and it has become extreme, the skin may be punctured with a lancet or drained by a small silver cannula (Southey tube)." Southey had not developed his procedure until after the reports of original followers of Bright. Osborne was the most conservative in recommending laxatives, avoiding them when there is already diarrhea, and cautioning against gamboges, jalap and cream of tartar, favoring Castor Oil and Magnesium Salts. Richard Bright used laxatives freely as part of the treatment of "inflammation", stating : *"Purgatives generally act well; the Elaterium in the case of Evans evidently gave much relief, and all the saline laxatives which unite a certain degree of diuretic power are decidedly useful. Amongst these I have found the Supertartrate of Potash (Cream of Tartar) the most efficacious."* P. Rayer was equally enthusiastic in the use of "depletion therapy" of which blood letting and laxatives were a part: "One sometimes gets a noticeable reduction and sometimes a disappearance of the dropsy by purging the patients twice a week with Sedlitz water (mixture of tartaric acid, cream of tartar and sodium bicarbonate) or Pullna water. (Both Sedlitz and Pullna are villages in Bohemia with mineral springs with high concentrations of sodium and magnesium sulfate) Cream of tarter has also given with good results in Senna tea. The dropsy has sometimes diminished through the use of drastic purgatives, by administering elaterium in a quarter grain dose at a time or at a higher dose administered in intervals of a few hours. I have tried colcynth mixed with extract of henbane. I have also tried gamboges administered everyday. In some cases, the dosage of scammonee or of gamboges can be raised." Osler as well as the earlier writers considered laxatives as diuretics in their ability to dehydrate the patient and so remove the edema. Osler was more selective in his use of laxatives, avoiding combinations of colcynth and henbane as well as Cream of Tartar in senna tea, not considering gamboges or scammonee.

Bleeding was an ubiquitous form of depletion therapy in the early nineteenth century and did not escape Osler's attention, "If uremic convulsions occur—from a robust strong man 20 ounces of blood may be with drawn." From Sir Robert Christison report in 1829, shortly after Bright's initial *Report of Cases* of 1827, are described seven patients that fulfilled Bright's criteria for renal disease. The fourth case, Murdock Campbell, 27 years old, a labourer and night watchman, may hold a record for the quantity of blood withdrawn, with a salutary result. The patient was bled initially 34 ounces, not the 20 ounces described by Osler, and as might be expected, "felt weak and faint." This was followed by 36 ounces and then cupping for 14 ounces, *"from which great relief was obtained and his abdominal pain and somnolence improved.."* An additional 40 ounces of blood were finally removed as well as application of leeches on several occasions as well as Potassium Supertartrate and other measures. Mr. Campbell most remarkably improved with the "urine becoming entirely free even of haziness when heated" This represented a total of 3.72 Liters of blood removed in a relatively short time! The patient was "kept in the hospital for security sake another month before being dismissed." Christison concludes, "I regret exceedingly that it was out of my power to learn what afterwards became of this man as he went to the island of Skye immediately after quitting the hospital."

Conservative Approach to Therapy

Richard Bright and Sir William Osler shared in not only depletion and antiphlogistic measures, but both also demonstrated a reasoned conservative approach to treatment. Osler: No remedies, so far as known, control directly the changes which are going on in the kidney" Richard Bright :"In those cases where, as in Bonham and Stewart, the kidney besides apparently having some morbid deposit, has become preternaturally hard, we can only employ palliative remedies: and if we could ascertain by well marked symptoms the existence of this state, probably the great advantage we should gain from the knowledge, would be in its restraining us from adopting those more active remedies, which would be apt to wear out the powers of life, without affording any permanent relief to the organs affected" This statement may even surpass the recommendations of Sir William: "Patients—should so regulate their lives as to throw the least possible strain upon heart, arteries, and kidneys. A quiet life without mental worry, with gentle but not excessive exercise, and residence in an equable climate should be recommended."

With regards to the treatment of persistent or albuminuria, Osler demonstrates his most conservative and cautious stance, "For the persistent albuninuria... we have no remedy of the slightest value. Nothing indicates more clearly our helplessness in controlling kidney metabolism than inability to meet this common symptom. Astringents, alkalies, nitroglycerin, and mercury have been recommended."

Mercurial Diuretics

Osler considers the use of mercurial diuretic, Calomel. "Many patients with Bright's disease present themselves for treatment with signs of cardiac dilatation ; there is a gallop rhythm or the heart sounds have a fetal character, the breath is short, and the urine scanty and highly albuminous, and there are signs of local dropsy. In these cases the treatment must be directed to the heart. A morning dose of salts or <u>calomel</u> may be given." In this instance Bright appears to be the more conservative: *"Still however, the cases which have proved most successful in my practice, have generally been those in which I have rigidly abstained from the use of mercury—there is one circumstance which most materially limits our power of employing it, and that is the violence and rapidity with which the ptyalism* (mercury intoxication) *often comes on."* Bright was the first to recognize the ease with which mercury intoxication can be produced in renal failure, *"inducing the gums and cheeks—to the process of ulceration and often passing into a state of gangrene."*

Exposure to Cold as an Etiological Agent
Alcohol and Scarlet Fever

In considering the etiology of the disease, Osler reports: "1) Cold. Exposure and wet is one of the most common causes. It is particularly prone to follow exposure after a drinking bout. 2) The poisons of the specific fevers, particularly scarlet fever." These were uniformly considered the etiological agent causing Bright's disease by Bright and is colleagues: cold, alcohol, and scarlet fever.

Bright summarizes his feeling, as well as that of all of his followers, in the introduction to Cases and Observations, Illustrative of Renal Disease Accompanied with the Secretion of Albuminous Urine published in 1836: "The first indications of the tendency to his disease is often hematuria—<u>scarlatina</u> has apparently laid the foundation for the future mischief—<u>intemperance</u> seems its most usual source; <u>exposure to cold</u> the most common cause of its development and aggravation."

The history of exposure to wet or cold and alcoholism was recorded in almost every case of Bright, Osborne, Christison, and Rayer. Bright's initial case John King, "a sailor till within the last four years, and was accustomed to take considerable quantities of spirits." Or consider Rayer's first case," Madame C., Spanish, very strong constitution—after having been exposed to cold and dampness, experienced etc. etc." Or consider Case 4 of Rayer: "Louise Caritte, 36, in good health, of a remarkable gay disposition, living in Paris for 17 years—attributed her edema to cold to which she had been exposed in her accommodations which were improperly shut up, located under the roof, and to a period in a low and damp spot in which her profession of a weaver forced her to spend the day." Rayer continues, "Much has been written on the abuse of alcohol, but it still hasn't been stressed enough, as one of its most serious and most dangerous effects, the kidney diseases which I shall treat here. When a doctor is called to care for people who have not been able to give up that deadly habit, he will carefully examine their urine, whatever the threat to their health of which they are complaining."

Dr. Osler, after accepting alcohol as a factor in the etiology of acute nephritis, relents and after discussing the possibility of toxic agents: turpentine, cantharides, pregnancy and extensive lesions of the skin, etc., states that Acute nephritis is particularly prone to follow exposure after a drinking-bout...but then modifying it, Alcohol probably never excites an acute nephritis."

Removal to an Equable Climate

Finally Osler concludes: "A change of air is often beneficial. Particularly a residence in a warm, equable climate. Or as he states later under the treatment of chronic Bright' disease: "A patient in good circumstances may be urged to go away during the winter months or, if necessary, to move altogether to a warm equable climate, like Southern California. There is no doubt of the value in these cases of removal from the changeable, irregular weather which prevails in the temperate regions from November until April."

However we find that Osler was not the first to recommend a change of venue for Bright's disease. Richard Bright himself in his Cases and Observations illustrative of Renal Disease Accompanied with the Secretion of Albuminous Urine in the Guy's Hospital Reports Vol 1 of 1936, "I have suggested the propriety of a residence in some more agreeable climate, but I have never had an opportunity of giving a fair trial to this measure, the disease being, unfortunately, most apt to occur in those who are least able to submit to the absence from business and the expense incident to a residence abroad...Perhaps, to give full effect to a change of climate, some decidedly southern abode should be chosen: and a residence in one of the more healthy of the West-India islands, as St. Vincent's would probably be beneficial." Bright at least was honest enough to admit the absence of a controlled study in this matter in that he had not had "opportunity of giving a fair trial to this measure."

Rayer in the Traite, indicates, "To that end the doctor will recommend living in a dry and temperate environment, in a flat with southern exposure, proper alimentation appropriate to the digestive system, daily use of ferruginous (iron) preparations and of a small quantity of good white wine. And in the case where later the dropsy will disappear, where the disease is reduced to a renal dysfunction of a disorder of urinary secretion, the patients could prolong their life by a continuation of the same regimen, by the habitual use of lukewarm aromatic baths, and by moderate exercise, if unfortunately the social class of most of them does not make it possible to undergo costly and long term continuous care." Sir William Osler could not better express more clearly his own conservative therapeutic creed any better...Again Osborne, quoted earlier from his 1838 volume On the Nature and treatment of dropsical diseases, has almost the same advice as that of Osler, "For those in affluent circumstances a resident in a warm climate cannot be to strongly recommended."

Osler with his acceptance of the earlier 19th Century's concepts combined with his conservative approach to medication follows the above advice on moving "to a warm equable climate, like that of Southern California." Expressed alternatively Osler observes, "Patients derive much benefit from an annual visit to certain mineral springs, such as Poland, Bedford, Saratoga, in America, and Vichy and others in Europe. Mineral waters have no curative influence upon chronic Bright's disease; they simply help the interstitial circulation and keep the drains flushed. With that emphasis on "helping the interstitial circulation", Osler again shows his acceptance of older underlying assumptions of the depletion therapy.

The "removable to an equable climate", whether Southern California in the case of Osler or St. Vincent's Island in the West-India Islands for Bright, or a "flat with a southern exposure" as favored by Rayer, all have as their underlying assumption that chill or cold are of etiological factors in the cause and can lead to aggravation of the disease. Avoiding suppressed perspiration with use of flannels to keep a patient warm is a similar example ploy. Osler went right along with these assumptions of an earlier period.

Subsequent Editions of the Principles and Practice

1916 Edition Edited by Thomas McCrae

Perhaps later editions of Osler's Text would edit out these echoes of the earlier century. A review of the eighth edition from 1916 edited by Thomas McCrae, 24 years after the original publication and used by my father in medical school promised "largely re-written and thoroughly revised" is thoroughly disappointing in this regard. Only minor changes were added to the Treatment of Bright's disease such as: 1) a single sentence was added to the last paragraph of the 1892 edition, to the effect that morphia is helpful in the management of the dyspnea of Cheyne-Stokes breathing as well as in managing the central nervous system manifestations earlier noted in the 1892 edition, 2) a paragraph on Surgical Treatment, citing the recently introduced operation of decapsultation of the kidney, a currently discarded form of treatment that has not sustained the evidence of time, and 3) the dangers of Pilocarpine were omitted in this later edition. In addition to dry or wet cups for relief of pain in the back or haematuria, the 1916 edition edited by McCrae also includes the Paquelin cautery. (a platinum point for use in cauterizing, hollow and filled with platinum sponge, through which a heated hydrocarbon vapor is blown, developed by Claude A. Paquelin a French phusician 1836 – 1905)

16th Edition edited by Sir Henry A. Christian, 1947

The last edition of Osler's *Principles and Practices of Medicine*, the 16th edition was edited by Sir Henry A. Christian in 1947. This was 31 years after the eighth edition from 1916 and 55 years after the original 1892 edition. The 16th edition under Christian is thoroughly edited and purged of therapeutic measures such as thyroid extract, Digitalis, "unless there is evidence of heart failure", and hot applications to and cupping of the loins. Exposure to cold and wet along with alcoholism were the major etiological factors considered by Bright, Christian, Rayer, as well as Osler in the 1892 edition. Christian in this 1947 edited edition modifies this opinion. "Exposure to cold and wet, included as a rule among causes, probably plays a part only through consequent respiratory tract infection; the same is true of burns, the effect on the kidney being indirect. Toxic agents, such as terpentine, mercury, arsenic, potassium chlorate uranium nitrate, .. (previously considered major factors by the earlier authors as well as Osler in the 1892 edition) of much interest in the production of experimental lesions in animal kidneys, scarcely plays any part in the natural disease in man." Bed rest continued to play an important part of treatment in 1947, but modified slightly, "Bed rest, so long as the urine contains rbc, casts, other than hyaline ones, and considerable albumin is our most effective therapeutic agent." Osler in 1892 was more direct, "The patient should be in bed and there remain until all traces of the disease have disappeared." About the only unchanged or unmodified dictum from the 1892 first edition of Osler's *Principles* is the familiar dictum, "A quiet life without worry with gentle but not excessive exercise, and resident in an equitable climate" and the equally familiar suggestion, "that a patient in good circumstances may be urged to go away during the winter months, avoiding changeable winter weather ... Patients derive much benefit from annual visits to certain mineral springs such as Poland, Bedford, Saratoga in America, but mineral waters have no curative influence in Bright's Disease. . This last phrase that Christian adds agrees with Osler in 1892 edition in that "Mineral waters have no curative influence upon chronic Bright's disease", but drops Osler's 1892 concluding phrase, "they simply help the interstitial circulation and keep the drains flushed." This 1947 edition of Osler "Principles and Practice" is probably the last text book of Medicine to use the appellation, Bright's Disease for the more currently used term glomerulonephritis.

Osler's Textbook Revisited 1967

Osler's Textbook revisited was published in 1967 and edited by Drs. A.M .Harvey and V.A. Mckusick;. This volume sets the historical aspect and reviews the circumstances of the writing of *The Principles and Practices of Medicine* and reprints the 1909 seventh edition of Osler's textbook, as this was the last edition that was written with the sole authorship of Dr. Osler. Each of the various disease entities are evaluated as to what additional knowledge was available currently in 1967, and in the case of Renal Diseases this was edited by Dr. Maurice B. Strauss of Boston, Mass. With regard to treatment, Dr. Strauss gives Osler credit for considering salt restriction, "As there is marked retention of chlorides, which seem to bear a relation to dropsy, salt should be withheld." This important caveat in the treatment of the edema of Bright's Disease did appear in the 1909 and subsequent editions of *The Principals and Practice of Medicine* but not in the original 1892 edition. Dr. Strauss quotes Osler's conservative attitudes toward treatment, *"No remedies, so far as known, control directly the changes which are going on in the kidneys. The indications (treatment) are: (1) to give the excretory function of the kidney rest by utilizing the skin and bowels, in the hope that the natural processes may be sufficient to effect a cure; (2) to meet the symptoms as they arise."* Dr. Strauss chose not to comment on Osler's therapeutic echoes of the earlier nineteenth Century that included many depletion and antiphlogistic measures. It is recognized that Dr. Strauss' review was to emphasize the prescience of Dr. Osler and the advances he detailed since Bright's original observations.

Finally Dr. Strauss trips over Dr. Osler's recommendation for the *"removal of 12 to 20 ounces of blood, if the patient was robust and full blooded, as had Richard Bright a century earlier"* as similar to the "custom of today when even frail and pale patients are bled daily of an ounce or so by white-coated technicians." This changes the emphasis from the ancient depletion mode of therapy to a current frenzy to establish a diagnosis with a plethora of laboratory data. Dr. Strauss does not comment on Osler's reasonable dictum recommending to a patient in good circumstances to go away during the winter months.

Edition of Osler's Principals and Practices 1986 Edited by Drs. Harvey, Mckusick,

The most recent edition of *Principles and Practice* in Osler's name from 1986, edited by Harvey et al. is a thoroughly modern Text, placing renal disease right at the beginning of the book, chapters 1-3, replacing the position of Typhoid Fever in all the previous editions. The first two chapters are devoted to physiology and electrolyte considerations. The third chapter mentions treatment briefly, discussing bicarbonate for acidosis and binders for elevated phosphorous, and of course dialysis and transplantation. Banished from this expurgated edition are any of the echoes of the early nineteenth century depletion therapies, but absent as well are any allusions to the humanistic and quality of life issues that came through in the 1892 through 1947 editions of Osler: "Patients should so regulate their lives *as to throw the least possible strain upon the heart, arteries, and kidney. A quiet life without mental worry, with gentle but not excessive exercise, and residence in an equable* climate." This 1986 edition of Osler's text likewise omits any similar humanistic references that had similarily been previously encouraged by Rayer: " *the doctor will recommend living in a dry and temperate environment, in a flat with southern exposure, proper alimentation appropriate to the digestive system,------and a small quantity of white wine."* Perfect for a Frenchmen! While I am glad this latest edition of Sir William Osler's text has finally absolved itself of calomel, strophanthus, strychnia, cupping wet and dry, cream of tartar, and bleeding etc, missing are the concerns of the patient's over all care and situation. Still why did it take so long to remove the shades and echoes of early nineteenth century therapeutic concepts in the treatment of Bright's Disease?

Summary

Certainly William Osler's recommendations for treatment of Bright's Disease have a tone of compassionate and humane understanding, as are the recommendations of Bright, Osborne, and Rayer which have been quoted. Under *Prognosis* of Chronic Bright's Disease, Osler remarks, "Chronic Bright's Disease is an incurable affection, and the anatomical conditions on which it depends are quite as much beyond the reach of medicines as wrinkled skin or gray hair." But intermixed with a non-pharmacological approach are distinct echoes of the depletion therapy, use of the skin and bowels and blood letting that was a part of the older authors, Bright, Christison, Osborne and Rayer. Osler did not recommend many of the concoctions that Bright and his colleagues used frequently. Bright was very fond of Dover's Powder, a combination of ipecac and opium, or as with the first prescription for John King, Mercury, Squill, and opium. Richard Bright may have considered these as well as Sulphate of Quinine with Squill, or Uva Ursi (bear berry) as tonics, *"it is as a tonic that the Uva Ursi is sometimes useful."* Rayer is much more varied in his use of medication that Osler never mentions: Horseradish tea, donkey milk, couch-grass tea, leeches to the rectum for GI complaints, colchicum wine, etc. Steven Peitzman has suggested that Osler's "therapeutic advice rested on medical tradition and the underpinning of authority rather than physiology or statistics." David Macht reviewing Osler's prescription writing noted that he used many drugs, "prescribing only chemical agents the physiological action of which had been sufficiently demonstrated." Macht pointed out that he "avoided combination of drugs and herbs that had mystic combinations of polypharmaceutical agents." This paper documents this comparison in the use of medication as compared with his predecessors. Macht considers Osler, rather than a therapeutic nihilist, as some have labeled him as "a pioneer in rational pharmacotherapy."

Therapy in part depends on the concepts of the etiology of disease. The early Nineteenth Century and earlier considered removal of noxious products by the skin and blood, necessitating phlebotomy, laxatives, leeches, baths, and methods to stimulate sweating as prime principles of therapy. Bright in his section on treatment outlines the rationale for depletion treatment. *"When the inflammatory attack comes on early in the disease, it is often overcome by very free depletion…Bleeding is a most important remedy with a view of restoring the healthy action of the kidneys; that is, with the view of removing what appears to be the chief source, if not of the disease itself, at least of many of its most alarming symptoms."* Christison was equally as direct, *"Treatment of the primary disease, (requires) rigorous antiphlogistic remedies."* Inflammation was the process to be concerned with. The definition of inflammation in the early nineteenth century may have been somewhat more vague than that used today. Fever and membranous appearance of the serum were important but also effusions in chest, heart, and abdomen pointed to inflammation and the primary therapeutic tool was depletion therapy in the form of phlebotomy, sweating or laxatives. Inflammation has taken on a broader significance recently being implicated in a wide variety of diseases, not unlike that in the early eighteenth century, being implicated in Atherosclerosis, as well as other conditions. Today we are attracted by the immunological causes of disease, including kidney disease and employ such methods as Steroids and Immunosuppresion as key to therapy. Will this stand up in the next 65 years, the time between Bright and Osler?

Osler and Bright both understood the limited knowledge of the basic underlying etiology of renal disease and strove for symptomatic relief of complications rather than radical cure. However echoes and reminiscences of the earlier nineteenth century armamentaria of laxatives, blood letting, cupping and efforts to stimulate the skin with pilocarpine and baths were listed by Osler perhaps in respect to past efforts at treatment. However in other chapters of *Principles* such as on Typhoid fever and later on in the text on Tuberculosis where over 75 pages are devoted to its consideration, echoes of the earlier eighteenth century practices are much less evident. With Tuberculosis, "spontaneous healing is an everyday affair—it is a question of nutrition, digestion and assimilation and making the patient grow fat." The surroundings are important and the use of sanitariums stressed. "No medical agents have any special action on the tuberculosis process peculiar." Sanitarium care with fresh air and purity of the environment and good accommodations and food were the norm for treatment of tuberculosis. The early nineteenth century depletion therapies played no role in either the treatment of Typhoid Fever or Tuberculosis.

Osler's textbook of 1892 did contribute newer information on the therapy of Bright's Disease as compared with that in the writings of the earlier Nephrologist. 1) The management of cerebral symptom such as seizures and delirium were no longer treated with leeches to the temporal area, but with chloroform or morphia. 2) Diet was considered with restriction of meat and salt, although milk was recommended.3) Blood pressure was considered, although that term is not used, Osler preferring *increased arterial tension.* Undoubtedly Osler knew of the work of Frederick Mahomed and Samuel Wilkes who carried on the Guy's Hospital tradition of studies in renal diseases, broadening the concept of Bright's Disease to include hypertension and vascular disease. Osler quotes Mahomed in the first edition of *Principals and Practice 1902,* in connection with, "in a case of scarlet fever it may occasionally be possible to avert an attack (of nephritis) the premonitory symptoms of which are marked increase in the arterial tension and the presence of blood coloring matter in the urine (Mahamed). An active saline cathartic may completely relieve this condition" This observation on treatment probably is of doubtful value. Osler was more concerned about too great a lowering of the "blood tension", preferring, "a happy medium (to) be sought between such heightened tension as throws a serious strain upon the heart and risk rupture of the vessels to low tension" For persistent high tension he recommended a light diet and nitroglycerine. Also considered for hypertension, more in line with the earlier nineteenth century concepts were occasional saline purge and "sweating promoted by means of hot air or the hot bath" The lack of adequate anti- hypertensive medications is apparent.

This paper details the modes of therapy that William Osler inherited from preceding authors from Richard Bright through Christison, Osborne, and Rayer. Remarkably Osler accepted rather uncritically the earlier 19th Century therapeutic practice of sweating, laxative, hot baths, bleeding, cupping, and mercury in the form of calomel, while in considering other diseases such a s Tuberculosis and Typhoid Fever, he was more circumspect and conservative. He does not label his treatments as antiphlogistic or aiming to produce depletion, but accepts them uncritically. Equally astonishing was the very slow progress in making changes in Osler's suggestions for therapy over the 94 years from the original 1892 edition to 1986 edition edited by A.M.Harvey, V.A. Mckusick et al. This applies to the humanistic comments to *"so regulate their lives* and *seek a residency in an equitable climate "* as well as to the therapies representing the baggage from the earlier nineteenth century. The genius of William Osler's textbook of 1892 was the organization of all disease entities into a systematic consideration beginning with Pathology, Symptoms, Diagnosis, Prognosis and finally Treatment. With regards to treatment for Bright's Disease, shades of this cumulative baggage of earlier nineteenth century practice were present perhaps to a greater degree than in his consideration of other diseases such as Typhoid fever or Tuberculosis where his usual conservative and compassionate approach predominated.

Afterword
David B. Levy

It is hoped that this modest contribution to the field of the history of medicine, with these included essays in the history of nephrology, will also make a positive contribution to the scholarly community which hopefully will enjoy and find this work, except the introductions, conducted during Dr Levy's retirement as represented in the enclosed essays, a welcome further addition to filling in some of the gaps in our knowledge and understanding of the evolution of the field of the history of nephrology and allied sciences

This volume is but volume 2 of a proposed 5 volume set. The first volume on *Music and Medicine* occupies a place of great importance in better understanding the *medical Humanities* which give the medical profession a cause and higher mission. This afterword on the Medical Humanities is included to try to show that each volume is not a separate unconnected volume from the rest of the set. Rather it is a vision of Humanistic medicine that inspires and gives coherence to the complete five volumes.

Hippocrates once remarked, "*where there is love of human beings there is also love of the art of medicine.*" Nietzsche, in the work, *Die Geburd Der Tragedie*, sketched out a vision of a holistic man of science in what he called Apollonian medicine, of a music-practicing Socrates. The physicians' prayer ascribed to Maimonides, but according to Dr Fred Rosner written in the 18th Century,[1] urges physicians to be sensitive, caring, with a service ethic, to enable the quality and longevity of life and eliminate pain and suffering. Unfortunately, the Nazis twisted Nietzsche's thought and gave birth to the opposite of the Apollean music practicing physician i.e. a Dionysian medicine of Nazi doctors who had not care, humanity, or compassion in their "cyclopic" drive to reduce human beings to lab rats and guinea pigs for cruel and barbaric medical experiments. Perhaps, as Holderin remarks in the poem Patmos, "where the danger is, there is the saving power too." Medicine can save lives but it can also be abused as the Nazis showed in their human experiments on victims of the Holocaust. Dialysis[2] and organ transplants truly do give extra years if not decades and longer to their recipients and that is indeed a "saving power too."[3] There is a distinction in the literature regarding however

---

[1] Rosner, Fred, "The physician's prayer attributed to Moses Maimonides," *Bulletin of the History of Medicine* 41 (1967), 440-454.

[2] Kaplan De-Nour, Atara, Dialysis and transplantation services in Israel, Israel Journal of Medical Sciences 9 (1973) 918-922.

[3] See Friedlaender, M.M, Kidney transplantation in Jerusalem, 1972-89, Israel Journal of Medical Sciences 28,1 (1992) 1-8.

altruistic kidney donation and those done for monetary compensation.[4]

In the 19th century, William Osler of Johns Hopkins University had a vision of medicine's social dimension to better and further the well being and common good of communities and secure the health parameters for each person to live a life in pursuit of liberty and happiness. Osler's favorite book, which he collected all editions of, was *Religio Medici*, or the Religion of Medicine, for Osler understood medicine was a calling, just as religions speak of callings, that required selflessness on the part of physicians to attempt to fulfill the mantel of such a field with the potential to do so much good.

Oliver Sacks brings particular sensitivity and care towards his discipline of neurology and care of his patients. His book *One Leg to Stand On*, which documents Sacks' own being a patient so that he better learned how to put himself in the shoes of others, allows Sacks to combine brilliant literary talent with a medical humanistic vision of genuine respect for all human beings and dedication to the scientific advancement to wipe out disease and illness within the methods of the medical profession. Not since William Carlos Williams, a poet and physician, who lived in Rutherford, NJ, had a medical practitioner been able to harness literary technique to be ministerial to a *Medical*

---

[4] Jotkowitz, Alan, A Jewish perspective on compensation for kidney donation, Assia - Jewish Medical Ethics 7,2 (2010) 13-19; Grazi, Richard V., Nonaltruistic kidney donations in contemporary Jewish law and ethics, Transplantation 75,2 (2003) 250-252.

Humanistic vision. In Sacks' work *Awakenings,* we see the social dimension of medicine as the main character physician invents a drug that allows patients in a catatonic state to emerge from their mental hibernation to awake and live life more fully, but when the government withdraws funding for the production of the medication, the patients tragically return to their catatonic slumbers. *Awakenings* is also a book about the awakening of the main character in Sack's story who is awoken to the understanding that life is with people in community and his former reclusive behavior is abandoned with the courage to ask a nurse out on a date, after he lived his life primarily occupied with his work and hobbies such as butterfly collecting. The main character undergoes like a butterfly a metamorphosis into an awakened state that life is worth living and we must make the most of our lives not to waste time and "cherish our days."

The example of Albert Schweitzer is a case in point of a physician with a vision of the Medical Humanistic ethical altruistic and selfless devotion to the well being of others. Schweitzer gave up a potentially prosperous career as a physician and/or a concert organist (he wrote a 2 volume set on the music of Bach) and instead opted to relocate to the then third world of Africa and offer medical help to underserved populations. It is reported Schweitzer dug the foundation for his own hospital with his own hands, donated his own blood, gave up his own coat to clothe the cold, selflessly devoted himself to wipe out the plague of malaria there. This represents a tincture of his boundless efforts to secure medical supplies and treatments for his patients. Albert Schweitzer was saint-like by putting himself at risk, and represents a physician who gave up everything in the realm of material comfort, (being an illustrious graduate of Harvard University that would allow any door to provide to him for securing his own wants), but rather chose to make a difference in the world of medical praxis with underserved populations in Africa. Schweitzer's calling was a radical ethic. He put his own private interests to the back burner and pursued his vision of the common good.

A physician should be well rounded like a Renaissance man. That means being familiar with all aspects of the Humanities. Literature gives us many ways in which to mirror the experience of illness as found in the short stories such as Thomas Mann's *Death in Venice* and *Magic Mountain*, Tolstoy's *The Death of Ivan Ilych*, or Dr. Conan Doyle's *Round the Red Lamp*. Authors like Treves, Francis Brett Young, A. J. Cronin, and Somerset Maugham have made use of their medical knowledge in fiction, and non-medical writers have done the same. Who can forget the masterly picture of locomotor ataxia in Kipling's story "Love of Women," or the harrowing account of cancer in Arnold Bennett's *Riceyman Steps*? Charlotte Perkins Gilman's short story, "*The Yellow Wallpaper*' lets us see the dangers of medical mistreatment in the area of psychology as representative of the confining and misogynistic ramifications of Victorian "rest therapy" for women suffering from post-partum depression. As Michel Foucault has brilliantly demonstrated in works such as *The Birth of the Clinic*, and throughout his oevre, power-knowledge regimes sometimes can harm innocent persons just as represented in the novel *One Flew Over the*

Cuckoo's Nest, where a lobotomy is performed on the main character. A novel of the philosopher and Nazi resistance fighter Albert Camus recounts the portrait of a selfless physician named Bernard Rieux in *La Peste*, who is the most ethical and moral individual in all of the protagonists of Camus' multi variegated literary works.

Medicine gives the chance to help give the gift of life, and that is so awesome and powerful that one may hope that the best and brightest go into this field, with the potential to extend quality and longevity of life and eliminate pain, with a commitment and calling to others . Such is the hope of the Medical Humanities, to make us better human beings, and more empathetic, compassionate, and ethical practitioners of the art of medicine and science.[5]

---

[5] Burks, Derek & Kobus Amy M., "The legacy of altruism in health care: the promotion of empathy, pro sociality and humanism," 10 February 2012 https://doi.org/10.1111/j. 1365-2923.2011.04159.

Bibliography

Papers Written While in Medical School (1949-1953)

1. Dissimilation of glucose-1 phosphate and of fructose 1-6 phosphate by isolate rat diaphragm and by cell free effluent from rat diaphragm: K.L. Zierler, R.I. Levy, and R. Andres. Bulletin of the Johns Hopkins Hospital, 82:7, 1953.

2. On the mechanism of action of alpha-tocopheryl phosphate with special reference to carbohydrate metabolism of striated muscle.

      a. Effect on the capacity of rat diaphragm to dissimilate hexose phosphate: K.L. Zierler, R.I. Levy, H.M. Anderson and J. L. Lillenthal. Bulletin of the Johns Hopkins Hospital, 92:32, 1953.

      b. Inhibition of insulin induced glycogenesis on isolated rat diaphragm. K. L, Zierler, R.I. Levy, J.L. Lillenthal. Bulletin of the Johns Hopkins Hospital, 92, 41, 1953.

Papers Written during Nephrology Fellowship with Dr. Gilbert H. Mudge (1955-1957)

3. The effect of acid base balance on the diuresis produced by organic and inorganic mercurials: R.I. Levy, I. M. Weiner, and G. H. Mudge. Journal of Clinical Investigation, 37: 1016, 1958.

4. Studies on mercurial diuresis: renal excretion, acid stability and structure activity relationships of organic mercurials: I. M. Weiner, R.I. Levy, and G. H. Mudge. Journal of Pharmacology and Experimental Therapeutics, 138: 96, 1962

Papers Written During House Staff Training or Medical Practice (1959 – 2002)

5. Renal failure secondary to ethylene glycol poisoning: R.I. Levy. Journal of the American Medical Association, 173, 1210, 1960.

6. Steroid blocking agents as diuretic agents: R.I. Levy. Sinai Hospital Journal, 10:110, 1961.

7. Serum sodium concentration: Facts of Fancy: R.I. Levy. Indian Medical Journal, 1962, (October).

8. Lipids of the kidney, Blood and Urine in the Nephrotic Syndrome: R.I. Levy, Fifteenth Annual Conference on the Kidney 1964.

9. Antibiotics and Digitalis Administration in Uremia : R.I. Levy. Editorial – Maryland Medical Journal, 13, 1964.

10. Ethacrynic Acid in Pulmonary Edema: R.I. Levy, A.I. Mendeloff, D. Turner. American Journal of Clinical Nutrition, 18: 20, 1966.

11. Studies in a Patient with Chyluria: R. I. Levy, A.I. Mendeloff, D. Turner. American Journal of Clinical Nutrition. 18:20, 1966.

12. Overwhelming Salicylate Intoxication in an Adult: R. I. Levy. Archives of Internal Medicine, 119, 1967.

13. Treatment of Hypercalcemia with Forced Saline Diuresis and Ethacrynic Acid. R.I. Levy, Proceeding of the American Society of Nephrology, 3rd Annual Meeding Washington, D. C. (Abstract) 0.40, 1969.

14. Clinical Spectrum of Lactic Acidosis. R.I. Levy, K. Dharmasena (Paper presented at Regional Meeting, American College of Physicians in Baltimore, MD, October, 1975.

15. Serum Chloride Analysis, Bromide Detection and the Diagnosis of Bromism: American Journal of Clinical Pathology, R.I. Levy, R.E. Wenk, Lustgarton, Pappas and Jackson. Vol. 65: 49, 1976

16. Ectopic ACTH, Prostatic Oat Cell Carcinoma and Marked Hypernatremia, R.E. Wenk, B.S. Bahagavan, R.I. Levy, D. Miller and W. Weisburger. Cancer, Vol. No 2, August, 1977.

17. Chyloperitoneum in a Peritoneal Dialysis Patient. American Journal of Kidney Diseases. Vol 38. No. 3 (Sept) 2001; pE 12.

Unpublished paper

Mozart and Medicine at the End of the Eighteenth Century R.I. Levy 1990 Presented at Sinai Hospital Lectureship, Baltimore, MD

Papers Written Following Retirement from Medical Practice, 2002

18. History of Sinai Hospital of Baltimore Maryland 1863-2009, Its Place in the History of Jewish Hospitals in America

19. William Osler's Mention of Basham's Mixture in the Treatment of Bright's Disease: Who was Basham and What was his Mixture

20 The Animal Chemists in the Circle of Richard Bright

21. Therapeutic Spectrum Available to Defining the Newly Recognized Clinical Entity: Bright's Disease

22. The Reception in Britain and on the Continent of Richard Bright's-Report of Medical Cases on Linking Dropsy, Coagulable Urine and Small Granular Kidneys as a Clinical Entity

23. A Garland of Ibids: the Use of Footnotes in the Medical Writings of Early Nineteenth Century Authors Who Established Bright's Disease a Clinical Entity

24. Sir William Osler: A Departure from His Reputation as a Therapeutic Conservative: The Treatment of Bright's Disease

25. Urinalysis as a Factor in the Establishment of the Clinical Entity of Bright's Disease in the Early 19th Century

26. *Pulvis Impecacunanhae et Opii*—The Powder and the Buccaneer, Thomas Dover (1660-1742)

27. Sir William Osler's View of Pierre C.A. Louis' Recommendations for Bleeding in Pneumonia. The Paradox of Calling Louis's Method Iconoclastic, yet Continuing his own Practice of Bleeding in Some Cases of Pneumonia.

28. The Doctor and the Newspaper Editor/Literary Critic: Correspondence between Logan Clendening, M.D. and H. L. Mencken, 1924 thru 1944.

29. A conversation Between Two Leeches Refracted in English Literature from Shakespeare to Wordsworth, Concerning Round Worms: Their History, Function and Contribution to Medical Therapy—Past and Present

30. Colour Indicators, Robert Boyle's *Experimental History of Colours,* Lignum Nephriticum (Presented at the Osler Society May 2010)

30. Nicholas Monardes, Guaiacum—The Holy Wood from the New World and the French Pox.

31. Chevalier John Taylor, J. S. Bach, George Fredrick Handel—Did the Chevalier Really Operate on both Bach and Handel for Cataracts with Disastrous Results?

32. William A. Marburg's Contribution to Sir William's Osler's Love for books and Libraries

33. Brahms and Billroth: The Musical Composer and Physician—A Musical Friendship

34. Diagnosis of Handel's Opthomological Complications: The state of Opthomology at the time of Musician Fredrick Handel in the area of cataract surgery

35. William Harvey's *De Motu Cordis*

36. Homer Smith's Philosophy of Evolution and the Evolution of the Kidney

37. A Tribute to John Konrad Hemmeter

www.ingramcontent.com/pod-product-compliance
Lightning Source LLC
Chambersburg PA
CBHW071248220526
45468CB00001B/41